"Carolyn Coker Ross is a leading authority in the use of integrative medicine for eating disorders and addictions. Her new book offers a compassionate and highly effective approach to treating individuals with these problems. She offers both expertise and hope in showing us possibilities for transformation and healing at the deepest levels."

—**Andrew Weil, MD**, author of *Mind Over Meds* and *8 Weeks to Optimum Health*

"*The Food Addiction Recovery Workbook* is an important, much-needed resource in the field of eating disorders. Carolyn Coker Ross once again blends cutting-edge science with clinical wisdom and compassionate, practical tools. I highly recommend this book!"

—**Jenni Schaefer**, author of *Goodbye Ed, Hello Me* and *Life Without Ed*, and coauthor of *Almost Anorexic*

THE
Food Addiction
Recovery
Workbook

How to Manage Cravings, Reduce Stress, and Stop Hating Your Body

---

CAROLYN COKER ROSS, MD, MPH

New Harbinger Publications, Inc.

Publisher's Note

Distributed in Canada by Raincoast Books

Copyright © 2017 by Carolyn Coker Ross
      New Harbinger Publications, Inc.
      5674 Shattuck Avenue
      Oakland, CA 94609
      www.newharbinger.com

Cover design by Amy Shoup

Acquired by Jess O'Brien

Edited by Susan LaCroix

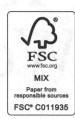 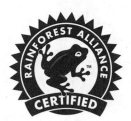

Library of Congress Cataloging-in-Publication Data

Names: Ross, Carolyn Coker, author.
Title: The food addiction recovery workbook : how to manage cravings, reduce
 stress, and stop hating your body / Carolyn Coker Ross, MD, MPH.
Description: Oakland, CA : New Harbinger Publications, [2017] | Includes
 bibliographical references.
Identifiers: LCCN 2017015522 (print) | LCCN 2017029227 (ebook) | ISBN
 9781626252103 (PDF e-book) | ISBN 9781626252110 (ePub) | ISBN
 9781626252097 (paperback)
Subjects: LCSH: Eating disorders--Treatment. | Eating
 disorders--Psychological aspects. | Nutrition. | BISAC: SELF-HELP / Eating
 Disorders. | PSYCHOLOGY / Psychopathology / Eating Disorders. | HEALTH &
 FITNESS / Nutrition. | SELF-HELP / Substance Abuse & Addictions / General.
Classification: LCC RC552.E18 (ebook) | LCC RC552.E18 R676 2017 (print) | DDC
 616.85/26--dc23
LC record available at https://lccn.loc.gov/2017015522

19 18 17

10 9 8 7 6 5 4 3 2 1   First Printing

Contents

Introduction

Everyone has heard someone say, "I'm addicted to chocolate" (or bread, or chips, or some other food). Generally, what people mean is that they like a food so much that it's hard to stop eating it. But an unknown number of people actually do find it impossible to stop eating certain foods. They feel out of control when they are around these foods, and crave them when they are not. This is now being called *food addiction,* and it is a very real problem in the same way that addiction to alcohol or illicit drugs is for some people.

In this book, you will learn more about food addiction and you will learn why it is not about the food. Food addiction could be called *eating addiction* because it's really about how you *use* food, and the very real consequences associated with how you use it. Out-of-control eating can cause obesity and feelings of shame, among other difficulties. Obsession with food can take over your life and create distance between you and those you love. You may find yourself so obsessed with food that it interferes with your work, and the body image issues associated with food addiction can keep you from doing the things you want to do.

In this book, for the sake of clarity, I will use the terms *food addiction* and *eating addiction* to mean the same thing. But as you learn more about this addiction, you'll gain a better understanding of why food addiction is not about food. If you struggle with food or eating addiction, this book will show you the path to recovery. While it may seem unimaginable now, you truly are capable of breaking free and reclaiming your life.

The reason food addiction may be more properly called eating addiction has to do with the question of whether or not it is really possible to be addicted to food. Unlike with drugs of abuse, we cannot be abstinent from food. You have to eat to survive. And there are many people (you probably know a few) who eat sugary, fatty foods regularly but don't seem to have trouble stopping or controlling how much they eat. While researchers and experts are clear that certain substances, such as cocaine and opiates, are addictive, there is still quite a bit of controversy about whether certain foods are addictive. It may be that, just as with substance use disorders, the substance is addictive only in a vulnerable person—for example, someone with a genetic risk for addiction. After all, there are people who drink or experiment with drugs who don't get addicted to drugs or alcohol. Now researchers are trying to understand whether people can be addicted to food and, if so, how this addiction resembles addiction to drugs and alcohol or how it is different.

Defining Addiction

Alcohol and drug addiction are specific in that they center on addiction to a substance. If you struggle with food addiction, this is what is called a *process addiction*. In other words, you may be addicted to or dependent on *behaviors* rather than *substances*. Process addictions can involve things like compulsive sex, gambling, or shopping; they can also involve restricting your food intake or bingeing (eating large quantities at one time). You may have difficulty stopping these behaviors and you may also get a sort of "natural high" similar to that seen with alcohol and drug addictions.

Any addiction—to food or to a substance—shares some common characteristics in that it is chronic, with numerous relapses. It involves compulsion to seek and "use" a behavior or a substance, and loss of control over how much and when you use or obsess about using. There is also a strong emotional component to addictions. For drug addicts, seeking their fix controls their lives—creating disruption in their relationships and difficulty with work and other normal activities. For food addicts, when your "food fix" is not available, you may feel panicked, angry, sad, or otherwise distressed (Koob and Le Moal 1997). There is an important difference in that so far, it is not clear whether food itself is addictive. You may be totally focused on certain foods as the cause of your addiction, just as a drug addict focuses on her drug of choice. While you may feel as if you are addicted to potato chips or chocolate, food addiction is fundamentally a process or behavioral addiction; it is not about food but about how you use the food.

Food addiction, like addiction to drugs or alcohol, often begins as a way to manage stress, turn up the volume on pleasant emotions (like happiness or comfort), or dampen uncomfortable feelings (like anxiety, anger, or sadness). It involves an unhealthy obsession with food. You feel distressed; you believe a certain food will make you feel better; you eat it; and it works: you feel soothed or relieved, if only temporarily. Your brain learns that you can get a quick fix, and the cycle of addiction begins. If you are a food addict, you may be using food to handle stress or to manage your emotions. Once you begin down this road of eating too much of certain foods that you obsess about, imbalances develop in your body and your brain that lead to food cravings—one of the symptoms of food addiction. This is exactly what happens with drugs of abuse. Again, not everyone who uses drugs or drinks or obsesses about particular foods becomes an addict. In this book, you will learn about the life experiences and genetic risks that may make you more vulnerable to food addiction.

In spite of the commonalities between substance addiction and food addiction, it's important to remember that with food or eating addiction, the behavior is the core of the problem. If you are using food to deal with either positive emotions or negative emotions, if food is your way of feeling comfort or escaping from stress—then it is your use of food that's the problem, not the food itself. Drugs are potentially addictive and, in many ways, eating is potentially addictive too—both affect the brain's pleasure or reward center. Anything you do that gives you a reward can potentially be abused and you can become addicted to it—whether it is food, sex, gambling, drinking, or any other activity. But if you focus only on eliminating the food you feel is responsible for your addiction, you will miss out on a deeper form of recovery. This deeper form could be termed a journey to discovery because so many people with addictions have never known who they are at their essence. For various reasons that will be discussed in this book, addicts tend to numb their feelings with their drug of choice and so miss this opportunity of self-discovery. You can recover by stopping your use of drugs or food or alcohol, but if you don't explore the deeper reasons why you use, why you became addicted in the first place, you will have only a superficial and fragile kind of recovery—sometimes called "white-knuckling it."

You've probably heard reports in the media that some foods (such as sugar) are physiologically addictive. Later in this book, I will discuss the research about whether food itself is addictive and talk more about the distinction between substance addictions and process addictions. For now, I encourage you to just open your mind to the idea that what you're addicted to is a particular kind of *eating*, because, unlike with drugs, you can't abstain from food. If you decide that certain *foods* are bad or wrong or "addictive," you will just continue in the same cycle of restriction, compulsion, and shame—the mindset associated with your obsession with food that has caused you so much pain and suffering already.

If you're reading this book, it's likely that you identify with the concept of food addiction. In the next chapter, you will have the opportunity to evaluate whether you suffer from food addiction and see what form your food addiction takes. This will begin to open a door to seeing all the ways in which the way you use food has affected your life.

PART 1

Understanding Food Addiction

You are beginning on a journey that will change your life in ways you can't fully imagine. Don't be afraid. I'll be with you every step of the way, holding your hand and directing you down the path you will follow. I commend you on the courage I know it takes to try to change your life. If you've been struggling with food addiction for some time, it may have affected many areas of your life—relationships, social activities, mood, physical health, and emotional well-being. Starting this journey may feel like a daunting undertaking. This book is here to break that journey into steps so that you don't have to feel overwhelmed. I have taken many of my patients on this type of journey before—for anorexia, bulimia, binge eating disorder, food addiction, and addiction to alcohol and drugs. This book will empower you to finally get back into the driver's seat in your own life. You will gain a lot of knowledge, but more than that, you will regain your sense of who you are.

The book is set up to allow you to take on what you are able to master a little at a time. I encourage you to reach out for support from your friends and from the eating recovery groups that are mentioned in this book whenever you need it. Remember, this is your personal journey to healing from food addiction. Don't judge yourself about anything in this book. This journey doesn't have to be finished in a certain time or in a certain way. Use what's here to support yourself in removing blocks, facing challenges, and learning new ways to deal with your life that allow you to free yourself from the hold food may currently have on you.

If you have picked up this book, you don't have to ask yourself if you're ready. You are! Turn the page and begin to make the changes in your life that you've been longing for!

CHAPTER 1

Are You a
Food Addict?

Jenn was in her mid-fifties when she first came to see me for her weight issues. Neither of her parents was overweight. She was an only child who had moved around a lot because her father was in the military. She was married, and although she and her husband had not been sexually active for many years, she still felt supported and loved by him. She was very physically active—swimming and playing on a women's softball team. Her history held one dark secret: she had been gang-raped as a college freshman and never told anyone.

When we discussed her relationship with food, Jenn became very animated. She was a self-described food addict. She talked about how her heart rate would increase and her mouth would water when she was in the chip aisle of the grocery store. She talked about trying to avoid going shopping because she knew she wouldn't be able to resist buying the large bag of chips that was her "downfall." But she also described her anticipation of getting the chips. She described the feeling as being like a drug addict going to score crack cocaine. She felt like a kid in a candy store—guilt-free and excited about her purchase. She sometimes felt the need to explain to the cashier why the bag was open: "I missed lunch today, so I'm starving!" When she got to her car, she would dig in in earnest. Before she knew it the bag was empty and her fingers were greasy and salty. She would lick her fingers and then try to wipe her hands on something in the car. She'd clean up the crumbs so her husband wouldn't know what she'd done.

Jenn described her shame and embarrassment after eating the bag of chips in her car in the parking lot. She felt like she had let herself down and wondered how she could have let herself eat the whole bag. But then the cravings would start again. She felt caught in a vicious cycle. She would think about the experience multiple times a day, beating herself up for giving in to the cravings. She sometimes went out of her way driving home to avoid any stores. She would make promises, then bargains with herself to keep herself from buying the chips. Or if she gave in to her cravings, she would promise herself she would eat just half the bag and then put them away. She also came up with punishments she would give herself if she slipped. Her eating felt completely out of control. Sometimes she would overeat or binge on other foods, thinking this would keep her from the chips. While much of her life was going well, this was a part of her life that felt miserable.

In the introduction, you learned about what food addiction is and what is isn't. Food or eating addiction relates to behaviors and thoughts that become obsessive and out of control and that have a detrimental effect on your life. These behaviors may include obsessing about certain foods, overeating or bingeing on certain foods, and being overly focused on your size or shape. People with an eating addiction may be thin, overweight, or obese. The common denominator among most people with this form of disordered eating is their obsession with food, and a desire to change both their eating behaviors and the effect that obsession with food and eating has had on their lives. In this chapter, you will be able to learn more about how you use food in your life and determine whether you have a food or eating addiction.

How Do You Know If You Are a Food Addict?

Since 2010, researchers at Yale University have been using the Yale Food Addiction Scale (YFAS) to identify people with food addiction. Using the same criteria used to identify people with substance use disorders, they have found that 5 to 10 percent of the general population test positive on the YFAS, including 7 percent of children tested. The YFAS also shows that food addiction is 15 to 25 percent higher in those who are obese. Even higher rates of food addiction are found in those who are seeking bariatric surgery or in obese individuals with binge eating disorder (30 to 50 percent). Binge eating disorder shares a number of characteristics with what is being called food addiction. Fifty-seven percent of people diagnosed with binge eating disorder also meet criteria for food addiction. In both disorders, people experience a lack of control over their eating, continued overeating despite negative consequences, and the inability to change their behaviors. Though there is some overlap between binge eating disorder and food addiction, there are also differences. People with food addiction tend to experience higher levels of poor self-esteem, depression, and difficulty regulating their emotions (Gearhardt et al. 2011a).

Use of the YFAS has allowed researchers to develop statistics to form a cohesive definition of food addiction. One of the markers that 100 percent of those taking the test answer yes to is "the desire to cut back or stop" their eating behavior. If you test positive on the YFAS, you likely have more intense and frequent food cravings than someone who tests negative. In fact, brain scans show high levels of activation in parts of the brain associated with cravings in response to food cues. In other words, when people with food addiction see highly palatable foods, their brains light up in a way that is different from people without food addiction. This pattern is similar to how the brain responds to drugs of abuse (Gearhardt et al. 2011b) or to hugging your child or doing any other pleasurable activity. If you have food addiction, you may be more likely to engage in emotional eating and may have an even more difficult time than someone without food addiction or other eating disorders being successful at maintaining your weight after dieting. Emotional eating can be defined as eating in response to emotional cues or eating to make yourself feel better or change your mood, as opposed to eating in response to being physically hungry.

Those who scored positive on the YFAS for food addiction tended to get more of their calories from fat and protein, rather than carbohydrates, as compared with those without food addiction. They also were more likely to have a history of child physical or sexual abuse (Meule and Gearhardt, 2014). Those who tested positive on the YFAS also had higher rates than the general population for depression and if obese, higher rates of attention deficit disorder. You may find this surprising, but as you'll learn in upcoming chapters, this association is all part of what is called *reward deficiency syndrome*, or RDS. RDS is a cluster of conditions that are thought to be the result of a deficiency in dopamine receptors in the reward center of the brain. With fewer dopamine receptors, individuals with RDS tend to be more vulnerable to addictions, attention deficit disorder, eating disorders, and other impulsive and compulsive disorders. In the exercise that follows, you can take a modified version of the YFAS to determine whether you have an eating or food addiction.

EXERCISE
Self-Test for Food Addiction

(Gearhardt et al. 2009)

1. How often do you find yourself consuming certain foods even though you are no longer hungry?

    a. Fewer than four times a week

    b. More than four times a week

2. How often do you worry that you should cut down on eating certain foods?

    a. Fewer than four times a week

    b. More than four times a week

3. How often do you feel sluggish or fatigued from overeating?

    a. Less than twice a week

    b. More than twice a week

4. How often do negative feelings about overeating interfere with important activities, such as work, recreation, or spending time with family and friends?

    a. Less than twice a week

    b. More than twice a week

5. How often do you experience physical withdrawal symptoms like agitation and anxiety when you cut back on certain foods (excluding coffee, tea, cola, or other caffeinated beverages and foods)?

    a. Less than twice a week

    b. More than twice a week

6. Does your behavior with respect to food and eating cause you significant distress? If yes, how often:

    a. Less than twice a week

    b. More than twice a week

7. How often do your issues related to food and eating decrease your ability to function effectively (daily routine, job or school, social or family activities, health issues)?

    a. Less than twice a week

    b. More than twice a week

In the past twelve months:

8. Do you keep consuming the same types or amounts of food despite significant emotional or physical problems related to your eating?

    a. Yes

    b. No

9. Does eating the same amount of food fail to reduce negative emotions or increase pleasurable feelings the way it used to?

    a. Yes

    b. No

To qualify as having a food addiction:

1. You must have answered "b" for *either* question 6 or 7, plus

2. You must have selected "b" or answered "yes" at least three times for questions 1–5 and 8–9 respectively.

List below the foods you have trouble controlling:

_____

_____

_____

_____

_____

If you were able to determine from the above test that you have a food or eating addiction, you may feel relieved to finally know why you've struggled so much with food and with your body. You may also feel somewhat overwhelmed to have a label put on you that you don't completely understand. The thing to remember now is that this recognition of the problem should not make you feel guilty or make you feel as if you should have been able to use your willpower to stop yourself from overeating. As you learn more about food addiction, you'll understand that it's not your fault. This realization should help begin to reduce the struggle you have in trying to control something that you feel powerless over.

In the next section of this chapter, you will learn about other characteristics of food addiction, which is a prelude to learning more about RDS, discussed earlier.

Characteristics of Food Addiction

Any addictive process has twin dragons driving the addictive behavior: impulsivity and compulsivity. *Impulsivity* is the tendency to act quickly without planning or thinking about consequences. Some people do recognize that what they are thinking of doing may be harmful, but the thrill or excitement they expect outweighs the risk. *Compulsivity* means that you are aware of the downside of the behavior but you feel drawn to do it anyway, possibly again and again. Factors that can lead to your developing impulsivity or compulsivity include genetics, the environment you grew up in, a history of psychiatric problems, and substance use disorders. If you tend to have compulsive behaviors, you may have performed those behaviors not so much for pleasure, but to reduce tension, emotional pain, or anxiety—such as overeating compulsively when you're upset, anxious, or stressed. If you tend to be more impulsive, you are more likely to use your behaviors for pleasure (not just relief from pain), at least in the beginning.

You may find, like Jenn, that the anticipation and rituals involved in seeking out your food fix are very pleasurable. Over time, your behaviors may feel less pleasurable and become more compulsive (you continue to do the behaviors being fully aware of the consequences, or actually feeling bad at the time you're doing the behavior). If you tend toward impulsivity, you may also notice that you underestimate or ignore the negative consequences of your behaviors. You may feel that the thrill or high you get from your preoccupations with certain foods and your behaviors related to these foods (bingeing, overeating, self-deprivation) are more important than the consequence you may suffer or the harm you cause. For example, you may say to yourself that you know if you eat that box of donuts, you won't feel good later, but you don't care about that enough to stop yourself.

There are different motivations inherent in each of these twin dragons. Impulsivity is driven by a desire to obtain pleasure, arousal, or gratification. Compulsivity is driven more by a desire to alleviate anxiety or discomfort (Berlin and Hollander 2008). Both involve changes in the executive function area of your brain, called the prefrontal cortex. The prefrontal cortex controls judgment, decision-making, the ability to "learn by experience," and the regulation of your emotions (Siddiqui et al. 2008). For example, if you've had a bad day at work, you may want to tell your boss exactly what you think of her. The prefrontal cortex will help you to use good judgment and inhibit this impulse so you can keep your job. However, in people with addictions, the prefrontal cortex is impaired in its ability to override impulses or control compulsive desires. These changes in the prefrontal cortex are what lead to impulsivity and compulsivity. If you are impulsive, you may just live and act from the present moment without regard to future consequences. If you're more compulsive, you may feel driven to use food to relieve emotional discomfort. Once you eat that food you're craving, you will feel a sense of temporary relief. There is some overlap between impulsivity and compulsivity, and some experts view them as opposite ends of the same spectrum. In the exercises that follow, you can determine where you are on the spectrum—more impulsive or more compulsive.

EXERCISE
Are You an Impulsive Person?

Circle the traits listed below that best describe you. The term "food fix" refers to the food(s) you are most preoccupied with.

1. I often do things without thinking.

2. I find myself saying things that I later regret.

3. When I think about my "food fix" it makes me feel tingly or excited or happy.

4. I don't plan my meals; I just eat whatever sounds good in the moment.

5. When I am bored, I tend to overeat or to eat certain foods.

6. I get upset over small things and tend to use food to calm myself down.

7. I often start a new diet enthusiastically but have trouble sticking with it.

8. If I were given a choice between eating one piece of chocolate (or other favorite food fix or comfort food) now versus waiting 20–30 minutes and having access to more of that food, I wouldn't be able to wait.

9. If I see or smell a food I like, I can't help but eat some.

10. Sometimes when I pass by a fast-food restaurant, I find myself driving through the drive-through even though I didn't plan to do that, and even though I'm not hungry.

If you identified with four or more of the above statements, you may have an impulsive nature. This may make it more difficult for you to do things that require planning, such as making long-term lifestyle changes. In the exercise below, you will be able to increase your awareness of how impulsivity affects your relationship with food.

EXERCISE:
How Does My Impulsivity Affect My Relationship with Food?

List below one way in which you find yourself being impulsive. (Jenn's example: *I get so bored at work sometimes that I can't wait to get off. I don't consciously think about stopping at the grocery story, but sometimes a billboard or an ad on the radio makes me think about my food fix.*)

_____

_____

_____

_____

_____

What thoughts, emotions, environmental cues (such as things on TV or the radio), or situations tend to trigger your impulsivity around food? (Example: *When there's a birthday at work and people bring in cake, I try to take just one slice, but find myself going back for more all afternoon.*)

_____

_____

_____

_____

_____

Based on the questions above, what purpose do you think your impulsive behaviors around food serve? (Example: *When I eat impulsively, it's the most excitement I have all day.*) I have listed some possible ideas for you to circle, or you can write in your own ideas.

1. Impulsive eating makes me feel excited or "revved up."

2. Impulsive eating gives me something to look forward to.

3. Impulsive eating really does give me my fix for the day. The food fix feels the same as alcohol feels for an alcoholic.

4. Impulsive eating helps me _____

5. Impulsive eating helps me _____

_____

Becoming aware of your impulsiveness and putting a small "stop" between you and your decisions may help you reduce the negative consequences of impulsiveness. Before you go to the refrigerator, imagine a mental stop sign or red light that allows you to take a moment before you do something you will later regret. If you are able to interrupt your impulse, you can check in with your body and ask yourself if you're really hungry, or ask yourself, "What am I hungry for?" Throughout the book, you will learn many different ways to reduce your impulsive behaviors related to food. Continue with the exercise that follows to determine whether you are more compulsive than impulsive, or whether you are both.

EXERCISE:
Are You a Compulsive Person?

1. When I see or smell my "food fix," I can't stop myself from trying it.

2. Once I start eating a food I like or feel I'm addicted to, I can't stop myself.

3. I eat to escape from my feelings.

4. I tend to obsessively think about what foods I'm going to eat that day.

5. Even if I've binged or overeaten the day before, I start planning my next binge the very next day.

6. I have specific rules and rituals around my eating behaviors.

7. I think about food a lot even when I'm not hungry.

8. I feel that food controls my life.

9. I worry a lot about my eating behaviors to the degree that it interferes with my daily life.

10. I know my eating behaviors are unhealthy, but I keep doing them.

If you identified with four or more of the above statements, you may have a compulsive nature. Compulsivity having to do with behaviors around food makes it difficult for you to stop doing the things you have identified as causing suffering in your life. Later in this book, you will learn more about ways to address this issue. For now, you can become more aware of when you repeat actions that are not in your best interest and how much time you spend thinking about food, your body, and eating. Answer the questions opposite to help increase your level of awareness.

EXERCISE:
How Aware Are You of Your Compulsivity?

1. List below behaviors that you engage in to relieve anxiety or other uncomfortable feelings. (Example: *After work, I sometimes feel so exhausted and yet anxious, I keep driving by the ice cream store on my way home from work and I can't stop myself from going in and getting a large dulce de leche ice cream, even when I'm not hungry.*)

   _____

   _____

   _____

   _____

   _____

   _____

2. How much of your time do you spend thinking about your next "food fix," worrying about what you're going to eat, planning your next binge, or feeling upset or disappointed about what you've eaten or fearful about your next binge? Estimate the time as a percentage, with 100 percent being all the time and 0 percent being never:

   _____

3. What purpose do you think your food fix serves in your life? (Example: *My work is so stressful and I don't feel appreciated there. Sometimes I feel so anxious by the end of the day, I just need something to calm myself.*) Below are some ideas of ways in which your food fix may be helping you. Circle the ones that apply to you and/or add some of your own.

   a. My food fix helps me numb out my negative feelings.

    b.   My food fix helps me to calm down from either positive or negative emotions that make me feel off balance.

    c.   My food fix helps me relieve tension or stress.

    d.   My food fix helps me _____

    e.   My food fix helps me _____

    f.   My food fix helps me _____

        _____

Good work! Learning to recognize your own compulsivity is the first step toward regaining control of your life. As compelling as food addiction feels, the fact is, you do have the power to choose your own actions. This book will help you learn how. It's important to remember that food addiction is not your fault. You can't control many of the causes associated with food addiction that we will discuss in this book, but you will learn about many things you can do to lessen your vulnerability to food addiction. Food addiction is not about willpower, and dieting to lose weight will not fix food addiction. In fact, it may make it much worse. However, as you learn more about what causes you to be obsessed with certain foods or preoccupied about your body size or shape, you will be well positioned to make the changes you need to make to recover.

In the next chapter, you will go deeper in exploring how you became a food addict. But first, it's important to understand the *arousal cycle* that you may have experienced when you think about, smell, or taste one of your favorite food fixes.

The Arousal Cycle

No one is born with a crack pipe or a cookie in her mouth. There is a process that evolves over time and begins with use, progresses to abuse, and finally escalates to addiction. For a food addict, it may start with something as simple as your parents using food as a reward for good behavior or using food to comfort you when you're upset. You may then start rewarding yourself with food when you've done something you're proud of or when you feel the need to celebrate. You may progress further to using food to help you feel better when you're down. Over time, food then becomes your primary coping mechanism for all sorts of situations.

If you have a food addiction, you may have recognized yourself in Jenn's story at the beginning of the chapter. One of the components of Jenn's food addiction is the *arousal cycle,* or how she reacts to certain foods. (Here, "arousal" refers to general stimulation, not specifically to sexual excitement.) The arousal cycle consists of three phases (Koob 2009):

- Preoccupation or anticipation phase: In this phase, you can't wait to get your hands on your food fix. You look forward to it with great anticipation.

- Getting high on your food fix: You are enjoying the experience of eating your food fix. Sometimes your food fix can put you into a state of excitement or into a trance-like state.

- Withdrawal or let-down phase: In this phase you are feeling low, disgusted, shameful, or guilty. You may also have some physical aftereffects of indulging in your food fix—such as bloating, digestive problems, joint aches, or generalized fatigue.

If you think back on it, you may notice that in the early stages of your addiction, you ate and obsessed about certain foods primarily because you loved the way your food fix made you feel. (This is the impulsive aspect of food addiction.) As time went on, your food fix may have been used more often to reduce anxiety, stress, or depression. (This is the compulsive part of the food addiction spectrum.) This is similar to what happens with other forms of addiction. When people first start using heroin, for example, they are feeling all the joys of the euphoria and escape that heroin use provides. In the next phase of the arousal cycle, their use increases. Over time, as they get more and more addicted—both physically and mentally—they will tell you that they are using to keep from getting sick. If they don't use, they become anxious or restless, they have low moods, or they have physical signs of withdrawal and severe cravings. In the latter stage of addiction, they want to use to avoid the pain of not having their fix, rather than for the joy and anticipation of the "high." In your own experience of food addiction, you may notice that one stage stands out more strongly than the others. For example, with nicotine dependence in smokers, the getting high phase is not that prominent. The third stage, however, is very noticeable. Nicotine addiction is one of the more difficult addictions to get over because of the negative withdrawal symptoms that many people experience—such as severe anxiety, irritability, and feeling just uncomfortable in their skin.

In the following exercise, you will have the opportunity to describe the different phases of your arousal cycle.

EXERCISE:
Your Personal Arousal Cycle

In the spaces below, describe your arousal cycle with your food fix. Include emotions, thoughts, judgments, or body sensations with each part of the arousal cycle. To help you get in touch with your arousal cycle, think of your last binge or the last time you got your food fix. You can also reread Jenn's story at the beginning of the chapter, which describes her arousal cycle.

1. Preoccupation or anticipation phase:

   _____

   _____

   _____

   _____

2. Getting high on your food fix:

   _____

   _____

   _____

   _____

3. Withdrawal or let-down phase:

   _____

   _____

   _____

   _____

What have you noticed about how your arousal cycle has changed over time? Did you get more out of one phase early in your food addiction than the others? If so, which phase is prominent for you now? Has your anticipation about your food fix changed? Describe the changes over time that you've noticed in relationship to your food fix.

_____

_____

_____

_____

_____

_____

_____

_____

_____

_____

_____

_____

Understanding the impulsive and compulsive nature of food addiction as well as the arousal cycle will help you increase your awareness of how you relate to your particular food fix, as you come to understand the component parts of that relationship. In the past, you may have dealt with your obsessions with food and with your body by dieting. In upcoming chapters, you'll learn why this approach should never be used again.

Consequences of Food Addiction

Just as for any addiction, there are consequences related to food addiction that impact your life and the lives of your friends and family members. People with food addiction often experience depression related to their eating behaviors. If you have a food addiction, you may be more prone to health problems, stress, difficulty sleeping, digestive problems, fatigue, and thoughts of suicide due to hopelessness about your food addiction. You may also have higher risks for high blood pressure, type 2 diabetes, high cholesterol, heart disease, and certain cancers. You may experience pain from arthritis in your joints if you are overweight or obese, and you may also have sleep disorders related to your weight. Many of these health risks are related to lifestyle more than to weight. You can be healthy at any size if you are able to be physically active and have healthy eating behaviors.

More than any medical risks, food addiction is psychologically debilitating. Thoughts about food, eating, your weight, or your size can take over your life and make you feel isolated, hopeless, and unhappy. Your food obsessions may cause low self-esteem, anxiety, or panic attacks. You may feel sad, irritable, or emotionally detached or numb. Your work performance may suffer and you may feel isolated from your friends and family members. Food addicts often avoid social events because of embarrassment about their eating behaviors. It's important to heal your food addiction to enable you to get back into the life you want. In the upcoming chapters, you will learn more about how to do just that.

Wrap-up

You may see your food addiction as an overwhelming problem. You may even have tried to address the problem by making promises to yourself or trying to avoid your food fixes completely. Usually these approaches work for a short time but not in the long run. For freedom from food addiction in the long run, you have to take a closer, deeper look at what's driving your addiction and understand that fundamentally, addiction is not really about a substance or a behavior—it's about something more. That "something more" is what you'll learn about as you read this book. In the next chapter, you'll learn more about the causes of food addiction.

CHAPTER 2

What Your Childhood Has to Do with Food Addiction

Chris's mother died of breast cancer when Chris, the younger of two children, was not even two years old. Chris's dad remarried one year later. Chris's stepmother helped keep the family together but was not very warm and nurturing. Some might even have described her as "cold." Chris's older sister took on the role of Chris's caretaker after their mother died, but she was only five years older and didn't always know how to handle Chris, who was a very rambunctious kid.

Chris began to turn to food out of loneliness and anger when he was in middle school. Even though he was a handsome kid, he often felt isolated and different from the other children. By the time he was in high school, his classmates were teasing him for being fat. His acting out in school also didn't endear him to his teachers, and he was kicked out of two different schools before he finished high school.

When Chris first came in for treatment, he was five foot eight and weighed almost 300 pounds. On questioning, he admitted that he binged on a regular basis—often eating two to three times as much as his friends. Pizza and steak, in particular, were his favorites. Chris did not understand why he continued to binge despite efforts to stop. He had also started drinking heavily, especially on the weekends—again out of loneliness.

Chris didn't date much but had one significant relationship that started when he was twenty and ended after five years. The relationship was chaotic and Chris knew it was not healthy for him. But he still obsesses about his ex-girlfriend, thinking that he let the "love of his life" go. When he thinks about her, he becomes either upset or hyperfocused on what "could have been." He has run into his ex from time to time and then texted her and had trouble not thinking about her all day. Sometimes his obsessive thoughts even interfered with his work. He started a new relationship two years ago but was very conflicted about it and was still texting his ex-girlfriend. He was afraid of getting too involved with his new girlfriend for fear that she would leave him, too.

In the previous chapter, you learned how to tell if you have a food or eating addiction, and about the underlying causes of food addiction. You also learned about how impulsive and compulsive traits affect your relationship with food, and you were able to explore your personal arousal cycle and the consequences of your addiction. In this chapter, you will learn about something called *attachment styles*. The famous psychiatrist Sigmund Freud designated the mother's importance (in a child's life) as "unique without parallel, established unalterably for a whole lifetime as the strongest love-object and as the prototype of all later love relationships" (Freud 1938). You can replace "mother" with "primary caregiver," father, grandparents, or adoptive parents who may have been the ones to raise you. What's important is that you form a bond with your primary caregiver that enables you to feel secure and safe to explore the world, to depend on people when needed, and to trust others with whom you are in relationship. This is the simple, straightforward explanation of attachment when it works as it should. However, for a variety of reasons, you may not have had the opportunity to form a strong, supportive relationship with your primary caregiver.

About now, you may be wondering what "attachment" has to do with food addiction. The way in which you formed, or did not form, a bond with your primary caregiver affects the way you see the world, yourself, and your future relationships. It also affects how your brain functions. If you were not able to bond well with your primary caregiver, this experience can predispose you to destructive coping mechanisms such as bingeing or compulsive overeating. It can also lead you to feel bad about yourself in general—and, in particular, to be dissatisfied with your body (Cash et al. 2004; McKinley and Randa 2005). This is exactly what happened to Chris because of his mother's death. Problems with attachment can make it difficult for you to regulate your emotions, and you may experience difficulty tolerating frustration or distress in your life. Most people with eating disorders say that they have difficulty tolerating strong emotions. They use food to avoid feeling or triggering strong emotions. They also use impulsive ways to manage their emotions (Corstorphine et al. 2007). Both impulsivity and difficulty regulating emotions are strongly associated with food addiction (Pivarunas and Conner 2015). Attachment difficulties can put you at higher risk for depression and anxiety. All of these consequences can lead to food addiction. For example, if you are depressed, you may gravitate toward using foods to soothe your mood. If you are easily stressed, again you may use food in an addictive way to deal with your frustration.

In this chapter, we'll look at the different types of attachment so that you understand how attachment works when things go smoothly within the family and also what happens when things don't go so well. With that background, you'll be prepared to take a closer look at how attachment problems can lead you to struggle with your mood, your relationships with other people, and your relationship with food.

Understanding Attachment

Infants bond with their primary caregivers by smiling, reaching for them, and making pleasing sounds, and by receiving responses to their upsets or their accomplishments (crawling or walking, for example). Young children give and seek affection and comfort from their primary caregivers and turn to them for help and support. The relationship with a primary caregiver continues to grow and strengthen over time as the child expresses happiness upon seeing his caregiver after a separation. This bond allows the child to explore the world on his own, keeping the primary caregiver as a secure base to return to when needed. If you bonded in this way early in life, as a teenager you were probably more focused on exploring the world on your own—acting more independent, becoming more autonomous, and starting to have relationships with peers that were close and intimate. These are all signs of healthy attachment.

What does attachment look like from the perspective of the caregiver? Caregivers must be sensitive to interpreting the signals that the infant or child sends out and respond in a timely manner. Caregivers must be available physically and emotionally to the child and must accept the child's needs willingly. If your mother or caregiver was abusive or spent more time on her phone or watching television than with you, or if she was very self-absorbed, you may not have been able to develop this bond. Perhaps your caregiver was ill, or addicted to drugs or alcohol, or had mental illness. Or perhaps you lost a parent when you were very young. Your caregiver may have felt uncomfortable trying to meet your needs (perhaps due to her own lack of parental bonding). The result of this unavailability is that, as a child, you may have come to feel that your needs would not be met, so you just detached from feeling any needs. Or you may have gone in the opposite direction—becoming clingy or whiny and difficult to soothe. If your mother was unavailable or rejecting toward you for whatever reason when you were young, you may have come to see yourself as unworthy or unlovable.

Caregiver Styles

With these basic dynamics in mind, let's look more closely at some of the particular attachment styles caregivers may have.

1. *The secure caregiver* is in tune with her child and responsive to his emotions and needs. This attunement leads the child to believe that his needs will be met.

2. *The tuned-out caregiver* is unavailable or self-absorbed. She is emotionally distant and more concerned about what's going on in her own life, often ignoring or being oblivious to the needs of her child.

3. *The inconsistent caregiver* is sometimes sensitive and sometimes unsupportive. She can be intrusive. You never know from one minute to the next whether you will get the person who interferes or tries to control your life, or the one who is sensitive and nurturing.

4. *The disorganized or terrifying caregiver* may ignore a child's needs, and her behavior can be frightening or even traumatizing. There is always a sense with this type of caregiver that you are not safe. She may be abusive or neglectful. Children with this type of caregiver sometimes spend time in the foster care system or an orphanage. There may be long separations from their parents. They may come from an unusually large family, or have a mother with a serious mental illness such as postpartum depression. This type of caregiver is much less common than the others but can cause more serious harm.

EXERCISE:
What Was Your Caregiver's Style?

Using the information on caregiver styles above, describe the type of caregiver you had growing up. Your caregiver may fit into more than one category, so use whichever traits best fit your experience. (Example: *My mother was very much the tuned-out caregiver. She was always at work, and even when she was at home, she worked in her office. Whenever I tried to get her attention, she would tell me to "entertain myself" or say that she was too busy to play with me—that she had more important things to do.*)

_____

_____

_____

_____

_____

_____

_____

_____

Attachment Styles

As a child, you formed your own attachment style in response to your mother or caregiver's way of relating to you. If your caregiver was generally available and sensitive enough to you, you trusted that relationship and felt secure in exploring the world and relating to others. This is called *secure* attachment. However, if your caregiver was unavailable, unpredictable, or overly harsh, you were left with a fundamentally *insecure* attachment. Without reliable, sensitive support from your caregiver, you would have found it difficult to manage your emotions or trust that you were safe.

As you might expect, your attachment style has a major effect on your relationships with other people, not only during childhood but throughout your life. Listed below are the ways the various attachment experiences may play out in relationships. These are characteristics you may experience in your own life as a result of your caregiver's particular attachment style.

1. If your bond with your mother or caregiver was secure, you are not likely to have difficulty forming and maintaining close relationships. You probably have healthy boundaries and a good deal of empathy.

2. If you had a tuned-out caregiver, you may tend to avoid close relationships or emotional connections because you subconsciously believe that your needs won't be met. You may be emotionally distant and rigid, hypercritical of others, and not accepting of other's differences.

3. If your caregiver was inconsistent, you're likely to be insecure. You tend to have a lot of anxiety or anger, always needing reassurance. You may try to control things in your own life and blame others when things go wrong. While you can be very charming, you may also be unpredictable.

4. If you grew up with a disorganized or terrifying mother, it may be relatively difficult for you to fall in love, and you may have great difficulty maintaining healthy relationships. Partners may accuse you of not understanding their needs. Your life may be chaotic. You may have an explosive temper, or have trouble trusting others even while wanting the security of a close relationship. People who have been raised by disorganized caregivers are sometimes misdiagnosed as having schizophrenia or autism spectrum disorder.

EXERCISE:
Identify Your Attachment Style

Reflecting on what you've learned, describe the personal characteristics you recognize in your life that are a result of the attachment style or the type of bond you had with your caregiver. You may have characteristics from more than one category. (Example: *I grew up in a very chaotic home. I never knew when I got home from school whether my mother would be happy and loving, or angry. She often took her anger out on us kids. It's hard for me to be in a relationship because I'm always so insecure—feeling like I'm waiting for the next shoe to drop.*)

_____

_____

_____

_____

_____

_____

_____

Building Secure Attachment in Adulthood

Clearly, there are many ways in which the bond between mother and child may be ruptured. However, it's important to know that two-thirds of babies from middle-class families have secure attachment (Hanson and Spratt 2000). Furthermore, a ruptured bond can be repaired or replaced. Attachment is a lifelong process, and even if, for example, you suffered the loss of your mother when you were young as Chris did, or for other reasons were unable to form a secure bond, you may have been able to attach to another caregiver. Whatever your situation, it is not hopeless. You can develop a healthy attachment style even in adulthood. According to a renowned attachment researcher: "Virtually all children—if given any opportunity—will become attached, but the quality of attachment varies widely" (quoted in Cassidy and Mohr 2001, 277).

Trauma and Attachment

Possible causes of insecure attachment include poverty, violence in the home, lack of support (such as having an absent parent or absent extended family), foster care placements, and marital conflict between parents. But one of the biggest risk factors for insecure attachment is trauma. Since trauma is so important when it comes to attachment, I'll discuss it in further detail here.

A traumatic experience is one that makes you feel threatened. If you've been traumatized, you may have experienced feelings of terror, helplessness, or extreme fear. Your body may have reacted to trauma with a rapid heart rate, fast breathing, trembling, dizziness, or other physical symptoms. Sometimes trauma involves a single event, such as a natural disaster or a death in the family. Or trauma can be longer lasting, with multiple events over an extended period of time, such as when you've been abused over the course of weeks, months, or years. If you were neglected while growing up, if your basic needs were not met, this too can be traumatic.

Trauma has a number of effects on your body. Experts believe that traumatic memories are "stored" in the body and can be triggered when you experience certain smells, tastes, textures, or sounds. Sometimes someone touching you in a certain way can trigger these memories. Or the memory may be triggered by certain foods or food smells. You may not be conscious of the association between these body sensations and your trauma until you actually find yourself in the middle of a response to a trigger, or having dreams or flashbacks. When this happens, you may feel as if the trauma is happening right then, as opposed to it being a memory from the past (van der Kolk 2005).

If you have a history of trauma, you may have also noticed that you are always on "red alert." You are easily stressed compared with other people and you have a difficult time calming down during times of stress. The stress, and your reaction to it, can lead to using food as a way to self-soothe or to numb yourself from your feelings.

How Trauma Affects the Brain

Insecure attachment and trauma have important effects on your brain. Experts used to think that trauma mainly affected the mind—that is, the more subjective experience of self, consciousness, and personhood. It is now clearer that childhood maltreatment has effects on the brain itself. Traumatic experiences actually change how the nerve connections in your brain develop. In cases of extreme neglect or trauma, they can even affect brain size (Insel and Young 2001; Perry 2013) Childhood trauma occurs at a time when the brain is developing very rapidly and is literally being sculpted by life experiences. Brain development involves the formation of connections between nerve cells. Your experiences with your primary caregiver are critical to how these connections form in the brain. So, when positive experiences with caregivers and secure bonding occur over and over again, those experiences lay down tracks that foster feelings of security and safety in the brain. If negative, stressful, or traumatic experiences are more common in your history, your brain has laid down tracks that lead to feelings of insecurity, shame, guilt, and self-doubt. Childhood trauma or abuse can show up at any age and in many ways. It can show up internally as depression, anxiety, borderline personality disorder, suicidal thoughts, or post-traumatic stress. Outwardly, it can be expressed as aggressive behavior, impulsiveness, delinquency, addictions, or hyperactivity (Teicher 2002). Fortunately, the brain has the ability to change and heal over time. This ability is called *plasticity*.

How Trauma Can Lead to Food Addiction

Trauma can lead not only to insecure attachment but also eventually to food addiction. If you are a trauma survivor, your brain has developed to help you survive by keeping you hypervigilant to your surroundings, always on red alert, always on the lookout for the next blow or the next chaotic moment. This may be one of the reasons why you turn to food or to alcohol, drugs, sex, or other behaviors: to self-soothe when you experience this feeling of tension. Your brain has prepared you to react quickly to threats through the stress response, but this same survival mechanism causes the release of stress hormones (adrenaline and cortisol) that don't let other parts of the brain develop, especially those associated with better judgment, impulse control, and other higher brain functions. As you can see, then, the survival mechanisms related to trauma can lead to impulsive behaviors or poor decision-making around food.

You may be starting to realize that you have used food to cope with your anxiety or insecurities that stem from the lack of a secure bonding experience. Sometimes people become attached to food as their only friend. Or food becomes their only experience of love or comfort in their lives. In the next exercise, see if your relationship with food fits any of the attachment styles you've learned about in this chapter. For instance, is your attachment to food chaotic, rigid, or inconsistent?

EXERCISE:
How Has Your Attachment Style Affected Your Relationship with Food?

Describe how you have bonded with food and whether that bond was created to fill a gap caused by insecure attachment with your mother or primary caregiver. Ask yourself what it is about your relationship with food or with certain foods that makes it addictive. (Example: *Jane's bond with food fits the same pattern she had with her mother in some ways. She tends to try to avoid using food for comfort but then she longs for or craves that comfort. Her relationship with food can be very chaotic. It's an on-again, off-again type of thing.*)

_____

_____

_____

_____

_____

_____

_____

If you have not had a healthy bond with a primary caregiver in childhood, this may be reflected in your relationship with food. However, that relationship can be changed. Sometimes, a child without a healthy bond with a primary caregiver may find a healthy bond with a teacher, therapist, other family member, or close friend. Or your spouse or partner may be the first healthy attachment you've experienced. This healthier bond can become a model for how a good relationship should be. You can use this model, then, to change your relationship with food.

Example: *Jane has a close relationship with her therapist that developed after the age of thirty. What she'd like to bring from that relationship into her relationship with food includes: 1) dependability (the ability to depend on herself to do what she says she will do with food); 2) presence (she'd like to be present for herself when she'm around food, in the way that her therapist always was present for her); and 3) calm (she'd like to be as calm around food as she felt when she worked with her therapist).* Describe below three things you can bring into your relationship with food that are modeled by any healthy relationship you have in your life.

_____

_____

_____

_____

_____

_____

_____

Now list at least one action you can take to begin to shift your relationship with food. (Example: *To bring more presence into my relationship with food, I will turn off the television when I'm eating and listen to calming music instead.*)

_____

_____

_____

_____

_____

Hopefully, you are gaining a better understanding of how attachment issues can impact your relationship with food and can lead to food and eating addiction. This awareness can only improve your relationship with food, which is not the enemy or the cause of the real problem you have with eating. It is important for you to learn about the root causes of food addiction because these underlying causes may also have an impact on other areas of your life. If you have attachment issues, those issues can affect your intimate relationships, friendships, and even work relationships. They can make it difficult to feel close to your children and siblings, and diminish your overall quality of life. Addressing those issues in the context of your food addiction can then spill over into these other areas of your life, improving not just your relationship with food and eating, but other relationships in your life as well.

So far, you've explored your attachment style and considered whether your eating issues might be related to attachment issues. In the exercise below, you'll pull all of these insights together to tell the story of your longtime struggles with food and eating.

EXERCISE:
Your Story of Food Addiction

Describe how you developed food addiction, beginning with your earliest food memories and moving forward to your present-day relationship with food. (Example: *I have a picture of myself when I was maybe three years old, with a cute little dress and white leather lace-up baby shoes. In each hand I'm holding a large chocolate chip cookie. After realizing I have food addiction, I've often thought of that picture and wondered, why two cookies? I couldn't have gotten them on my own. Why would my mother have encouraged me to have more than one cookie? I remember lots of family events during which I was encouraged to taste special foods. My mother showed her love for her family by cooking these foods. By eating them, I showed her that I loved her back. I remember I was forbidden to eat certain foods once I started gaining weight as a child. I was put on my first diet when I was five years old. As I grew up, I overate any time I felt at all insecure or unloved. I continued dieting until I was in my fifties, when I finally got fed up with always being unhappy with my weight. When I think back on the cycle that started my food addiction, what I remember is being given too much (two cookies!), learning that food was a way to communicate love, and then, when I got fat, being deprived of the foods I'd been taught to love.*)

_____

_____

_____

_____

_____

_____

_____

_____

_____

_____

_____

_____

_____

_____

_____

_____

_____

No matter what your personal story of food addiction is, you should continue to remind yourself that, as in the example of the little girl with two cookies, there were many factors that led to your developing this issue. Give yourself credit for taking the step to begin a journey to recovery. And remind yourself that any journey of importance (as this one is) takes time and patience. You didn't develop food addiction overnight, and it won't change overnight. But with each step, you will get closer and closer to your end goal of freedom from your obsessions around food and your body. You're well on your way!

Wrap-up

In this chapter, you learned about attachment styles with your mother or primary caregiver and how those may impact your mood, your ability to be in relationships with others, and your relationship with food. Your early experiences with your caregiver helped shape even the size and function of your brain. Food addiction is fundamentally about the need for love. If there has been a shortage of love in your life, you may have turned to food to fill the gap. The good news is, you can find other ways to bring love into your life, and you can heal your relationship with food.

CHAPTER 3

The Biological Roots of Food Addiction

Peter was clearly in distress when he first came to my office. He was frustrated by his inability to lose weight and had multiple health problems including diabetes, sleep apnea, and high blood pressure. He had recently been diagnosed with depression. He told me both his parents were obese and his father was a recovering alcoholic, as was his grandfather. His younger brother struggled with addiction to prescription painkillers and had been diagnosed with attention deficit disorder.

Peter was a successful businessman, and he felt in charge of many aspects of his life, so he could not understand why he had no control over his eating. When there was a birthday party at work, he would find himself sneaking into the staff lounge to eat the remainder of the cake. At home, once he opened a bag of cookies, he had to finish it. He was ashamed and embarrassed by his eating habits and worried about his health. At thirty-two, he now weighed over 300 pounds. He felt he was at his wits' end and desperate to end his obsession with food.

In chapter 2, you learned how your childhood—including your attachment pattern and any history of abuse or trauma—may have led you to develop an addiction to eating and an obsession with food. In this chapter, you will dig deeper to understand how those childhood experiences may have affected your brain in ways that explain why you, like Peter, have difficulty controlling your impulses, dealing with cravings, or managing food obsessions. For many people, the problem begins even before birth, with a genetic vulnerability—that is, one that runs in the family. That tendency toward food addiction can then be worsened by changes in your brain chemistry and factors in your environment, including life stress, difficult relationships, the particular kinds of foods you eat, and even the advertising and media messages you're exposed to.

Food addiction, like other eating disorders, involves genetic, biological, neurochemical, and psychological causes along with the social ones. This chapter will discuss what we know about the causes of food addiction, and the science that backs it up. When you understand how food addiction develops, you are in a better position to overcome it.

Understanding Reward Deficiency Syndrome

Food is a source of pleasure for most people, and the source of pleasurable sensations originates in a part of the brain called the *dopamine reward center*. Dopamine is the brain chemical responsible for feelings of pleasure and reward. Anything that provides pleasure affects the dopamine reward center. Normally, the brain's hard-wiring works in your favor, motivating you to repeat activities that are life-sustaining by connecting those activities to feelings of pleasure or reward. If something feels good you want to do it more. This explains why sex and eating are generally pleasurable: they perpetuate the survival of the human species. However, this mechanism can go awry.

First, for people without food addiction, eating normal amounts of food provides enough pleasure, and overeating occurs only on occasion (Thanksgiving, for example). But if you have a food or eating addiction, you may not feel the same amount of pleasure when you eat normal quantities of food, or when you eat foods that are not your "food fixes"—that is, those foods that you crave and have difficulty controlling. Food addiction may be explained at least in part by changes in the function of the dopamine reward system.

Second, even eating that isn't really about survival at all (eating to nourish your body) can be driven by the reward-equals-survival dynamic. When you use food to provide comfort or to numb yourself from emotional pain, this behavior locks into the same mechanism that drives you toward life-sustaining activities. But in these instances, it's the need for comfort or relief from emotional pain that drives you to overeat. You may feel like you're craving a certain food when, in fact, you are craving a certain feeling or lack of feeling (numbness) that you're using food to provide. Once again, the result is that you are obsessed with eating, and you may binge on foods that modify your emotions.

Researcher Kenneth Blum described a syndrome he called reward deficiency syndrome (RDS) (Blum et al. 1996; Blum et al. 2011), defined by difficulty experiencing feelings of pleasure or satisfaction. RDS involves a failure in the brain's dopamine reward system. Specifically, people with RDS have abnormally low levels of dopamine D2 receptors. If you have RDS, your brain has a harder time "detecting" the pleasure signal carried by dopamine, leading you to want to "turn up the volume" by doing more of the thing you hope will bring pleasure (Stice et al. 2009a). Low D2 receptors in the brain may make you more prone to emotional eating and to bingeing. Interestingly, the number of dopamine D2 receptors goes down as your weight goes up (Wang et al. 2012; Wang 2001), reinforcing the tendency to overeat.

Low levels of dopamine receptors may result not only in food addiction but in an entire cluster of disorders that involve addictive behaviors, impulsivity, and compulsivity. RDS can be implicated not only in compulsive overeating but also in alcoholism, drug abuse, smoking, attention deficit disorder (ADD), compulsive sexual behavior, and pathological gambling. It can even be related to antisocial personality disorder, conduct disorder, and aggression (Blum et al. 2013).

Underlying dopamine regulation issues may explain why many people with binge-type eating disorders (and food addiction) have a higher risk for another addiction, such as alcoholism. This propensity is related to specific genes common to both (Shinohara et al. 2004). You may quit one addiction (such as alcohol) only to find yourself binge eating and obsessing about food. Some people have weight loss (bariatric) surgery and then develop an addiction to alcohol, sex, gambling, or drugs (Blum et al. 2012). If you've been obese enough to qualify for weight loss surgery, RDS may be the root cause of your constant cravings and compulsive behaviors. Until it is addressed, you will have a hard time staying abstinent from addictive or impulsive behaviors (Blum et al. 2011).

How Reward Deficiency Syndrome Can Lead to Food Addiction

Let's look more closely at how RDS can develop into full-blown food addiction. Dopamine is important in your motivations and in your choices of what you eat or overeat. The sense of pleasure associated with your food fixes is directly related to the amount of dopamine released when you think about, smell, or eat particular foods (Small et al. 2003). Certain types of food are especially rewarding—typically those that are high in sugar, salt, or fat (or all three). These foods are called "highly palatable"; they are highly stimulating to your brain (Volkow 2008). If you think your love of certain foods is all in your head—it is. It's in the pleasure molecules of dopamine released by your brain.

If you have RDS, your brain's response to these triggering foods may be different than the response of someone without the low dopamine levels present in RDS. These foods affect you more strongly. If you crave chocolate, for example, your brain will light up at the taste of chocolate, or even while seeing a picture of chocolate (Stice et al. 2009b; Stoeckel et al. 2008). This response is not as strong in those who do not have RDS (Rolls and McCabe 2007). People with food addiction are predisposed to find more pleasure than those without food addiction when they eat highly palatable foods. This predisposition can lead to problems with bingeing, cravings, and weight gain.

Binge-type eating behaviors stimulate the release of dopamine in the brain. If you are obsessed with food or if you see, smell, or eat highly palatable foods, dopamine is released in your brain cells, making you want to eat more of this pleasure-giving food (Hernandez and Hoebel 1988). This dopamine hit perpetuates compulsive overeating (Noble et al. 1994). In animal studies, overeating of highly palatable foods (high in sugar and fat) is what triggers food addiction–like behaviors (Johnson and Kenny 2010).

Even the *expectation* of eating one of these highly palatable foods can cause dopamine release (Wang et al. 2004). If you have food addiction, just driving to the grocery store or walking down the cookie aisle and thinking about getting your favorite cookies will activate dopamine release—even before the cookie goes into your mouth. Once dopamine is released, it may be much more difficult to interrupt your desire to eat these highly palatable foods. These brain changes in response to foods high in sugar and fat mimic brain changes seen in drug addicts and alcoholics (Avena et al. 2009).

The same events in the brain can also lead to cravings. When dopamine is released, you may experience a desire for food that you interpret as "hunger," when in fact you are not physically hungry at all (Wang et al. 2004). People without RDS usually eat when hungry and stop eating when full. Their brains and bodies work together to give them feedback about physical hunger. But when you have RDS, highly palatable foods lead to the desire (as opposed to need) to eat when you are not physically hungry—simply because the brain craves a dopamine fix. Animal studies show that sugar may have effects on the brain's dopamine reward system similar to those seen during drug craving (Pelchat et al. 2004; Spring et al. 2008). Over time, use of food to help your brain produce more dopamine will backfire in the same way as chronic use of any substance, and this can result in uncontrollable cravings (Blum et al. 2014). While there have been many books and media reports written about how addictive certain foods (especially sugar) are, it's important to recognize that the addiction isn't caused specifically by the food but by RDS. RDS makes your brain more likely to react to these highly palatable foods in an addictive way—causing cravings, obsessive thoughts, and loss of control.

The tendency to gain weight is yet another important difference between people who have RDS and people who don't. Animals with low numbers of dopamine receptors gain more weight than animals with normal dopamine receptors, even when they are fed the same high-fat diet (Huang et al. 2006). This finding suggests that people with RDS are more likely to gain weight even when they have the same diets as those without RDS. Perhaps you've had the experience of watching your best friend eat a large piece of chocolate cake and knowing she won't gain a pound, while you will. Some people can "eat anything they want" and not gain weight while others can't. That reality is explained by differences in how their brains function. In the exercise below, see if you can determine whether you have RDS.

EXERCISE:
Do You Have RDS?

Circle the number of the items below that apply to you. Then grade your self-test using the key at the end. (Adapted from RDS Quiz by Kenneth Blum.)

1. My favorite hobby is chess.

2. Playing poker is more fun for me than playing chess.

3. I enjoy being immersed in a good book for hours.

4. I enjoy high-risk or adventurous activities.

5. If I had a choice between getting a small reward now or waiting to get a bigger reward later, I would choose waiting for the bigger reward.

6. Given the choice between getting a small reward now or waiting for a larger reward, I prefer not to wait. I want it now.

7. Most people describe me as having a calm personality.

8. Most people describe me as having an excitable personality.

9. At work, coffee is not vital to my ability to complete work.

10. At work I could not get my job done without coffee.

To score your test, add up all the positives for even-numbered questions (2, 4, 6, 8, and 10). If you marked 1 to 2 of these questions as positive, you may have a mild version of RDS. If you marked 3 to 5 even-numbered questions as positive, you are highly likely to have RDS.

Learning about RDS can help you understand why some things are harder for you than for other people. A better understanding may help relieve some of the suffering you've experienced in constantly trying to change your impulsivity and compulsivity, and feeling as if you're getting nowhere. If you understand that some of these behaviors and traits are related to your RDS, you can begin to accept that and then find ways to work with the cards you've been dealt, instead of working against them. Later in the book, you'll learn strategies to make the most of the brain you have. You will learn about how diet, social support, and other changes you can make can improve your brain's function and help reduce the impact of RDS.

What Causes Reward Deficiency Syndrome?

Understanding the causes of RDS can help you feel less guilty about your eating habits and begin to see how to overcome your addiction. RDS is the result of both genetic and environmental influences. You may have been born with low levels of receptors, or you may have experienced childhood trauma, neglect, or abuse that decreased the number of dopamine receptors as your brain was developing. Listed below are some of the causes of RDS:

- Genetic predisposition that may have been passed down from parents with similar impulsive, compulsive, and addictive issues

- Prenatal conditions—mothers using alcohol and drugs, and malnutrition in the prenatal period

- Malnutrition—poor diet due to poverty, low-calorie dieting, food allergies, or food sensitivities that disrupt your ability to absorb nutrients

- Severe or ongoing stress

- Heavy and prolonged use of drugs of alcohol

- Childhood trauma, abuse, or neglect

Not everyone who has RDS has the genetic changes in dopamine receptors. However, if you have a genetic deficiency in dopamine receptors and function and you also have any of the other causes listed above, you have a 74.4 percent risk of developing some type of obsessive, compulsive, or impulsive disorder during your lifetime (Blum et al. 2014). About 67.6 percent of obese individuals have the genetic variant associated with RDS (Blum et al. 2000). If you are a person with any of these vulnerability traits and then you unknowingly overstimulate your dopamine center, this can trigger addictive behaviors with food, and can also lead to further impairment in dopamine function (Bello and Hajnal 2010).

Let's examine the causes of RDS in more detail.

Genetics

If you have severe or multiple problems related to reward deficiency (compulsive or impulsive behaviors such as addiction and others mentioned earlier), your condition is likely to have a genetic cause. Blum's research led to the identification of a specific gene that is present in 73.9 percent of obese people who also have a substance use disorder, compared with only 23 percent of obese people who don't have a substance use disorder (Blum et al. 2011). The research explains why many individuals with an eating addiction and obesity may also be addicted to drugs or alcohol: the common root cause for both is RDS. If you carry the gene for RDS, you won't experience as much pleasure from eating highly palatable foods and will be more likely to gain weight (Stice et al. 2010). This likely explains the familial, genetic nature of RDS that you saw in Pete's story.

EXERCISE:
Your RDS Family Tree

In the genogram opposite, identify relatives who you think may have—or had—RDS. (A downloadable version of this diagram is available at http://www.newharbinger.com/32097.) Refer to the list of impulsive, compulsive, and addictive behaviors and personality disorders earlier in this chapter. List any that are obvious to you or that parents or relatives have told you about. In the bottom box, put your name and note whether you have food addiction, obesity, a substance use disorder, ADD, or whatnot. The two boxes above yours would be for your mother and father, and then the boxes above your mother would be her parents, and so on.

You may be able to see from your family tree that your food addiction has a strong genetic component.

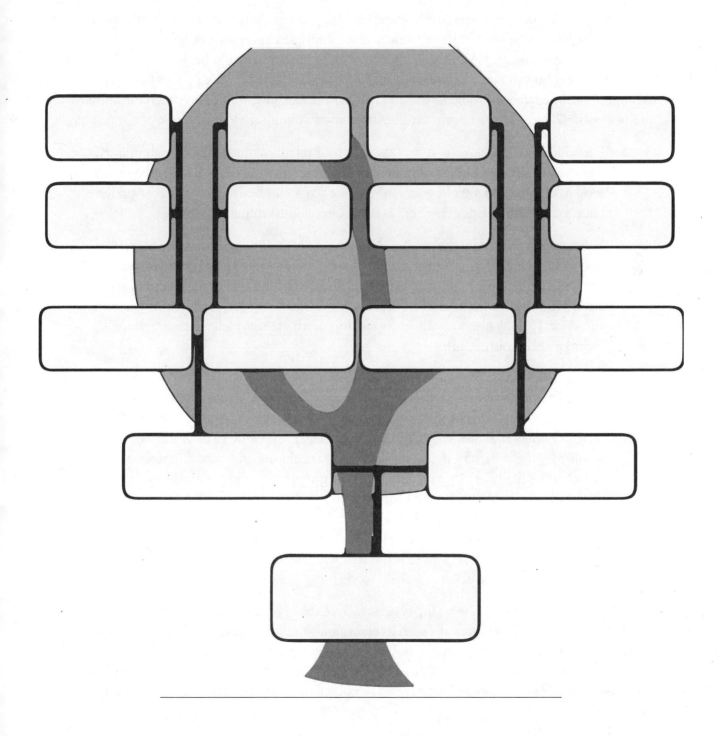

Environmental Factors

Reward deficiency problems may be inherited, but the environment can markedly increase your risk for RDS or make you more likely to have multiple expressions of RDS (for instance, compulsive overeating and ADD, or addiction to both food and alcohol).

Environmental influence begins even before birth. Prenatal factors can affect your risk for having reward-deficiency problems like food addiction. Because studies on pregnant humans are not possible, most of the relevant studies have used animals. Below are some of the results:

1. Diet during pregnancy: In animal models, feeding rats a diet that was high in fatty, sugary, and salty snacks during pregnancy and lactation predisposed their babies to food addiction and weight gain, an increased risk of obesity, and a higher preference for high-fat foods (Bayol et al. 2010; Ong and Muhlhausler 2011).

2. Substances ingested by the mother during pregnancy: Prenatal exposure to alcohol and drugs (including nicotine) may increase one's risk for RDS. For example, prenatal alcohol exposure has been well documented as a cause of fetal alcohol spectrum disorders, which include depression; anxiety; cognitive, attentional, and behavioral problems; and difficulty dealing with stress (Hellemans et al. 2010; Behnke and Smith 2013).

3. Exposure to stress: Stress is a major environmental factor contributing to changes in the brain that could lead to RDS. Both prenatal stress and early life stress can increase the risk of developing an eating disorder, addiction, and obesity (Su et al. 2016; Thomas et al. 2009; Taige and Glover 2007). Exposure to early life stress can result in more difficulty managing stress and regulating emotions throughout life, as well as a predisposition to mood disorders, impulsivity, and compulsivity. (Enoch 2011; Warren et al. 2014). Not everyone who experiences early life stress develops food addiction, drug addiction, or ADD. The effects of even severe childhood abuse or neglect can be reduced by strong family and peer relationships that foster resilience (Enoch 2011). This tells you that while some factors in your environment can cause problems, others can help to keep the brain in balance.

You may have been born with the genetic factors that predispose you to RDS, or you may have experienced early life stressors such as emotional trauma, or you may have been exposed prenatally to stress, or to drugs or alcohol, or to a poor maternal diet—all of which can cause RDS—or perhaps you experienced more than one of these things. Use the exercise below to identify environmental causes that may have contributed to your RDS and your obsession with food.

EXERCISE:
Your Environmental Factors for RDS

List any environmental factors that you have experienced or that you know your mother experienced either while she was pregnant with you or after your birth. I have listed some ideas to get you started.

1. My mother experienced a great deal of stress when she was pregnant with me because of:

   a. a natural disaster

   b. a death in her family

   c. divorce or marital conflict

   d. domestic violence

   e. addiction to drugs or alcohol

   f. a shortage of food

   g. _____

   h. _____

   i. _____

   j. _____

2. When I was very young, I experienced the following stressful or traumatic events:

   a. I did not have enough food to eat.

   b. I experienced a major loss in my life.

   c. I was adopted.

   d. One or both of my parents were drug addicts or alcoholics.

   e. I was molested.

   f. I was neglected.

   g. I was physically or emotionally abused.

   h. _____

   i. _____

   _____

Knowing more about your risk for RDS and the impact of life events on your current behaviors will help you to understand why you may have had more difficulty with food and body image issues than others. Later chapters will help you learn new ways of addressing these underlying causes of food addiction.

Growing Up in a Family with RDS

While there is a dearth of research studies on children of food addicts, there is some information that suggests that growing up in a home in which other family members have RDS can make you more prone to food addiction. Researchers know that in terms of weight or body mass index, about 25 percent of your weight can be explained by environmental factors and 25 to 75 percent is explained by genetics (Segal et al. 2009). As you read on, keep in mind that RDS encompasses a host of different disorders—from heavy smoking to drug addiction to food addiction and obesity.

Animal studies show that if children are exposed to cigarette smoke after birth, they are more likely to become obese as adults and to become drug or food addicts—a factor that may be explained by changes in the dopamine reward center (Pinheiro et al. 2015).

Your family's approach to food and eating can have a huge effect on your own eating patterns. For example, having family dinners with your children just three times a week can lower their vulnerability to obesity by 12 percent and disordered eating by 35 percent (Hammons and Fiese 2011). If you didn't routinely eat dinner with your parents, it stands to reason that you would have more problems with eating and weight. We know that children as young as nine years old show addiction-like eating behaviors due mainly to being "taught" to prefer certain (highly palatable) foods over other foods (Martin-Soelch et al. 2007). If you grew up in a family in which you were exposed to a diet high in salt, sugar, and fat, you are more likely to view those foods as preferable to fruits and vegetables, and to consume them in excess. Your parents' attitudes toward smoking and other substance use can make a difference, too; parental substance abuse has been found to increase a child's risk for overeating, obesity, eating disorders, and substance use disorders (Felitti et al. 1998). Children exposed to nicotine before birth also have an increased risk for obesity (Toschke et al. 2003).

Another very important predictor of overeating is your mother or primary caregiver's attitude about feeding you. If your mother tended to tell you not to eat certain foods, offered you food when you got upset, restricted your food and fat intake based on your weight, or made lots of negative comments about food, you would be more likely to engage in emotional eating, to overeat, and to gain weight (Bergmeier et al. 2015; Rodgers et al. 2013).

There is mounting evidence of the impact it has on children to grow up in a home in which one or both parents are alcoholics or drug users. The Adult Children of Alcoholics organization (www.adultchildren.org) clearly states that growing up in a dysfunctional household can lead to children feeling isolated and socially awkward. As a protection, many adult children of alcoholics become people pleasers and alcoholics themselves. They personalize criticism, are fearful of abandonment, and feel like victims throughout their lives. As you can see, there are various ways in which growing up with family members who have reward-deficiency problems can make you more likely to develop RDS yourself.

EXERCISE:
The Effect of Your RDS Family on You

Check off the traits that apply to you:

☐ My mother (father) always talked about how fat she (he) was even when her (his) body size had not changed or she (he) had lost weight.

☐ My mother (father) constantly made negative comments about her (his) body.

☐ My mother (father) made lots of comments about which foods were bad and which were good.

☐ I was put on a diet at an early age.

☐ I have trouble expressing or even being aware of my emotions.

☐ I have a very judgmental view of my body and myself.

☐ I sometimes overeat and don't know why.

☐ I often feel guilty if I stand up for myself rather than giving in to others.

☐ I have suppressed my feelings about the bad things that happened to me because I don't think it really matters.

☐ I am in relationship with someone with a drug or alcohol addiction or a food addiction.

If you identified with three or more of the traits above, you can see how your family may have unwittingly contributed to your eating addiction. It is important to recognize that that contribution didn't just come out of the blue. There is a genetic component, and there are also many environmental factors that can turn your RDS genes on or off. When you put the entire picture together, it should help you feel less guilty, embarrassed, or ashamed about your behaviors, your cravings, and your urges.

Food and Mood

Clearly, there is a strong connection between brain chemistry and eating behaviors. So it's not surprising that emotions play a major role in food addiction, too. You may have noticed that you overeat when you are depressed or anxious or stressed. This is referred to as "self-medicating"; essentially, the stress or unpleasant feelings are the "problem," and eating is the "medicine" that makes you feel better. People who are addicted to drugs or alcohol use these substances the same way: to try to manage negative emotions. If you have depression, anxiety, or bipolar disorder that's poorly treated or untreated, this can contribute to your being out of control with food.

The catch, of course, is that you cannot actually be abstinent from food the way you can from drugs or alcohol. Since it's not an option to stop eating entirely, it is helpful to look very closely at the particular ways in which you may be using food to self-medicate. Understanding the links between eating and mood can help you strategize effectively about healthier choices.

If you are obese, you are at higher risk for depression during your lifetime (Simon et al. 2006). When there is a deficiency or imbalance of dopamine in the brain, you may experience negative feelings such as anxiety, anger, low self-esteem, or difficulty coping with stress that you self-medicate with food or other substances or behaviors. When you eat sugary or high-fat foods, your brain not only releases dopamine but also releases internal *opioids*, leading to a reduction in feelings of stress and an uptick in mood (Fullerton 1985). While dopamine is related to the feelings of craving and wanting a certain food, opioids produced in the brain give you the actual pleasure from eating.

You can look at eating (from the feel-good standpoint) as having three stages: First you think about eating something and begin to crave it. Then you take action or are driven to get the thing you want. Both of these stages are related to dopamine production, as discussed earlier. The third stage is feeling satisfied and taking pleasure in what you are eating. This stage is governed by the production of opioids in the brain. Opioid production is part of the reward cycle; opioids simply make you feel better, at least in the short term. In the exercise below, you can explore your use of food to manage your mood.

EXERCISE:
Do You Use Food to Help You with Your Mood?

Check off the statements below that apply to you.

- ☐ I crave my food fix most when I'm angry or upset.

- ☐ I crave my food fix when I'm anxious or depressed.

- ☐ I find food very soothing.

- ☐ Sometimes I eat so much of my food fix that I become drowsy or fall asleep.

- ☐ I can actually feel myself calming down when I eat my food fix.

- ☐ Sometimes I don't even realize I'm upset about something until I realize I've over-eaten my food fix.

- ☐ I eat sometimes because I can't sleep.

- ☐ When I am sad, weepy, or down in the dumps, eating certain foods helps me get through the bad times.

If you checked off more than four of these symptoms, you probably use food on a regular basis to help you deal with your mood or with anxiety. Later in this book, I'll offer strategies for coping with emotions more effectively. If you have a history of a mood or anxiety disorder such as major depressive disorder, bipolar disorder, generalized anxiety disorder, or panic disorder, you may want to talk with your doctor to make sure your mood disorder or anxiety disorder is not making your food addiction worse.

Dieting Only Makes Things Worse...
and So Does Abundance

Animal studies on eating behaviors have highlighted something very important that is also seen in humans: While sugar appears to have addiction-like effects on animals, it is not the *exposure* to sugar itself that leads to addiction. Instead, researchers found that giving animals sugar, *then depriving them of sugar,* is what leads to cravings. When animals are deprived of their sugar solution for part of the day, they will binge on it when it is returned. After they no longer have access to sugar, the animals experience withdrawal-like symptoms similar to those seen with drugs of abuse. When deprived long-term, the animals that are offered drugs instead of sugar will become addicted to alcohol, cocaine, and methamphetamine at a higher rate than those animals that were not sensitized to sugar first (Avena et al. 2009).

For humans, just as for animals, it's depriving yourself of highly palatable foods that sets you up for cravings. Restricting highly palatable foods causes stress that then leads to relapse and binge-like eating behaviors (Bassareo and Di Chiara 1997; Teegarden and Bale 2007). This is the story you know. Dieting doesn't work, and deprivation itself is what makes diets so unsuccessful.

You may have heard that one of the issues contributing to the increase in weight problems in many developed countries is the abundance and availability of food (Volkow and Wise 2005). Fast-food restaurants used to be few and far between. Now, food is in your face all day long—with commercials on television and the radio, and billboards and magazines constantly telling you to eat this and that, and to supersize it.

This ease of access to food is not in itself the problem. The problem is that it can trigger the desire to eat at inappropriate times, to eat when you're not physically hungry, to eat more than your body needs, or to eat certain types of food for emotional comfort. This accessibility forces you to constantly check yourself and inhibit the desire to eat. This is harder for people who have low D2 receptors or RDS. If you have low receptors, the part of your brain that deals with impulsivity, emotional regulation, and the ability to make sound decisions may be impaired, making it harder for you to resist food cues and triggers that make you want to overeat. Just being exposed to food cues such as commercials can activate the part of your brain that motivates you to eat and causes cravings. When your brain is activated from food cues, dopamine is released—making you feel better even before you eat and motivating you to eat more. *This is especially true when you've deprived yourself of foods you want or like.* As you can see, dieting in an environment of food abundance just sets you up for failure.

Leveraging Your Brain Power to Overcome RDS and Food Addiction

When it comes to food addiction and other reward-deficiency problems, your brain may be a big part of the problem, but it's also a key part of the solution. Understanding RDS can help you overcome it using the power of the more rational parts of your brain. If you struggle with eating addiction, you may equate success with having the willpower to avoid overeating your trigger foods. When you actually learn more about how the brain controls eating behaviors through the dopamine reward system, hopefully, you will recognize that willpower is not always equal to the power of the brain chemicals that actually control your desire to eat or overeat.

Let's look at it from another viewpoint. The dopamine reward center is located in the part of the brain called the *mesolimbic* area. This part of the brain is triggered by positive and negative experiences (Ikemoto and Panksepp 1999). This is the part of the brain that deals with emotions, learning, memory, and motivation. It is also involved with personality traits such as thrill seeking, extraversion (being outgoing), and impulsivity (Bardo et al. 1996; Depue and Collins 1999; Cardinal et al. 2004). When you have a bad day and the first thing you think about is wanting to eat something, you are reacting to your emotions and acting from the mesolimbic brain, or "emotional brain." The same goes for when you find yourself in front of a box of doughnuts and can't stop yourself from eating them—you are motivated by powerful emotional urges or cravings, and your response to these emotions is automatic: eat, eat, eat. At the point in time when you begin to overeat or binge, you are truly not thinking clearly, because that would require that you use a different part of your brain—the *prefrontal cortex.*

The prefrontal cortex is the brain's executive thinker. This part of the brain is able to develop and carry out goal-directed behaviors, sustain attention on a project, make plans, and engage in problem-solving. It's your "rational brain." When you are emotionally upset, if you are able to recognize the desire to binge as part of the more primitive "emotional brain" that lacks control, you may be able to use your "rational brain" to interrupt the behavior and not simply react by eating. In the next chapter, you will learn more about how your emotions can often take over and run the show, and future chapters will provide you with skills you can use to take control of your behaviors. For now, it is important just to be aware of when you are in your "emotional" (mesolimbic) brain, versus the prefrontal cortex (your "rational" brain).

It is definitely hard to make the transition from "emotional mode" to "rational mode," and much more difficult if you have RDS. But over time, and with practice and help from what you'll learn in this book, you will find yourself more capable of consciously making the switch and taking control of your eating behavior. In the exercise that follows, you can plan some strategies to practice making this shift.

EXERCISE:
Shifting Your Brain

In the exercise below, identify situations when your emotions have "taken charge" with food. You can use previous binges, cravings, or obsessive thoughts about food. For each situation, write one action you can try to make the switch from your emotional brain to your rational brain. What would you tell your emotional brain in order to get it to calm down and be open to making this transition? The emotional brain is like a toddler in the middle of a tantrum, so be as creative as you can to help that part of your brain accept the need to act more rationally. Making this switch is like tamping down a fire that has already started in your brain, so the earlier in the process you can pour water on the fire, the more likely you will be to put it out.

Example:

Situation: *At the grocery store, I'm going down the cookie aisle and see my favorite cookies.*

Action I can take to shift my brain: *To avoid bringing a whole bag of cookies home, I can go to the other area of the store and purchase two cookies to take home with me.*

Why I would want to take this action: *I know if I take the bag home I will eat it all. If I buy the two cookies, I don't have to depend so much on willpower.*

Situation: _____

Action I can take to shift my brain: _____

_____

Why I would want to take this action: _____

_____

Situation: _____

Action I can take to shift my brain: _____

_____

Why I would want to take this action: _____

_____

Situation: _____

Action I can take to shift my brain: _____

_____

Why I would want to take this action: _____

_____

_____

It is important to know that natural reinforcers (events that increase the feeling of pleasure or reward) have the potential to increase dopamine release in the brain. For this reason, taking positive actions to shift from emotional responses to more mindful responses to cravings and obsessions about food, if done on a regular basis, can increase dopamine release and thereby reduce the impact that RDS has on your behavior and obsessiveness about food. Meditation, spiritual acceptance, love of others, physical activity, and participation in recovery groups are examples of natural positive reinforcers (Blum et al. 2015). Brain recovery will be discussed in more detail in part 3 of this book.

Wrap-up

It's very likely that your struggles with food addiction are rooted in RDS. Both your inherited brain chemistry and your life experience can set you up to feel obsessed with food and have difficulty regulating your eating. Emotions play an important role as well. Both dieting and overabundance of food can make the problem worse. In later chapters, you will learn specific things you can do to help heal your brain and improve its ability to provide you with the brain chemicals, such as dopamine, that you really need. While you can't always change your past or the genetics you were born with, in this era of intensive research on the brain in medicine, we are learning so much about the brain that shows you don't have to be stuck with the brain you have now or the brain you were born with. Don't despair—there are things you can change in your lifestyle that will change your brain, your mood, and your relationship with food!

PART 2

Healing from Food Addiction

In part 1 you learned about food addiction and how early life experiences, stress, genetics, and a personal or family history of addiction to drugs or alcohol could predispose you to having food addiction. You also learned about the importance of understanding reward deficiency syndrome as the underlying cause of food addiction. I hope that part 1 also enabled you to recognize that food addiction is not your fault, and that just using more willpower or trying to stick to diets will not enable you to gain control over the obsessive thoughts about food, the fears about weight gain, and the embarrassment and shame that accompany food addiction behaviors.

In part 2, I will lead you through three chapters that get you ready to begin the process of healing from food addiction. In these chapters, you will find a road map for the journey to healing that you are just beginning through the Five Levels. You will also learn more about your body and some of the hidden reasons you may crave certain foods, as well as what you can do to diagnose these hidden causes and to treat them. In the last chapter of part 2, you will learn how to break the hold that food has on you by detoxing your mind and your body. Working through part 2 of this book will prepare you to succeed in the plan for recovery from food addiction that's laid out in part 3.

CHAPTER 4

The Five Levels of Healing from Food Addiction

When I first met Lisa, I was bowled over by her big personality. She was vivacious and outgoing. She appeared very confident and spoke her mind whenever given the chance. Lisa was in her thirties, married to her high school sweetheart. She was a very successful executive in a large bank. She had a five-year-old daughter who was the love of her life.

The only glitch in Lisa's self-described wonderful life was her obsessive thoughts about food, her secret middle-of-the-night binges, and her ballooning weight. In public, she was a "picky eater," but in private, she couldn't control her overeating. She sometimes made herself sick from eating too much. She would then compensate for her binges by putting herself on a strict diet, but it never seemed to work; she didn't lose weight, and she was still obsessed with food. She felt ashamed of her eating behaviors and worried that she would pass her problems with food and with her body to her daughter, who was already starting to notice that Lisa never sat down to eat a meal with her.

Lisa felt disconnected from and dissatisfied with her body. In the process of working on her food addiction issues, she was able to identify that her binges on sweets late at night represented the comfort and safety that she didn't have as a child. Being molested by a neighbor when she was five years old marred her childhood. This traumatic experience led to her always feeling unsafe, as if she had to be on red alert both for herself and for her young daughter, whom she constantly worried would suffer a similar experience. When she binged on cake or cookies, she felt insulated from the anxiety or stress of constantly questioning herself or being afraid for her safety.

At times, Lisa felt completely numb when it came to thoughts about her eating or her size, but she was troubled nonetheless. She knew she was not able to express herself fully and that she held back at work and at home from being the truly free-spirited and joyful person she wanted to be. Her daughter reminded her of herself before the abuse, and she wanted to go back to being that happy and carefree person.

By this point in your life, you have probably realized that dieting over and over again has made your obsessions with food and eating worse—or at least has not made them any better. This is because when you focus on dieting, on food, or on the number on the scale, you are not addressing the underlying issues driving your addictive behaviors around food. In order to truly recover, as Lisa eventually did, you must come to a deeper understanding of the problem. In this chapter, you will begin to do this by learning about the Five Levels of Healing from food addiction. Tackling the core issues may sound daunting, but you can do it, and the rewards are considerable. Over time, you will become less obsessed with food, more comfortable making food choices, less prone to shame-based eating behaviors, and more forgiving of yourself when you slip up. You will be more able to accept your addiction for what it is—a pattern of emotionally driven eating that has its roots in a genetic condition and that "flowered" because of your childhood, your relationship with your parents, or experiences of stress and trauma in your life.

If you have any thoughts left in your mind that just losing weight will stop your obsessive thoughts about food or your body, this chapter should enable you to finally leave those behind. If you have any fears that you will just get fatter and fatter if you don't stay focused on what you eat or what you weigh, what you learn in this chapter will help you let go of that, too. This concern is understandable, but it's an example of unhealthy, diet-based thinking. You can develop a more healthy and comfortable relationship with food and with your body.

At the end of the day, what most people truly want is to be able to express themselves fully and without fear of judgment. It's natural to be concerned about what other people think, but consider this: fear of being judged is really about your own judgments of yourself. This chapter will help you understand what it means to be true to yourself. You'll learn to turn away from your inner critic and instead listen to your inner wisdom—the wise part of yourself that will guide you with kindness and gentleness toward reaching the goals that are right for you.

The Five Levels of Healing are your guideposts along the way. They will take you step by step through the stages that anyone who truly wants to heal at the deepest level possible must go through. Lisa's journey to healing using the Five Levels will help you understand how to begin your own journey and how to see it through to the end. The end is not a defined point in time. Rather, it is a measure of your progress. When your life is driven by your true desire to share who you are with the world, not by using food to fill a void that cannot be filled with food, you'll know you have arrived. The goal of learning about the Five Levels is for you to be able to identify things that no longer work for you, change old beliefs that don't belong in your life, address the behaviors that cause so much shame and guilt, and release toxic memories and patterns that are leftovers from the past. Working through the Five Levels will empower you to find true happiness and peace of mind.

Level 1—Stopping Superficial Behaviors

As discussed in previous chapters, bingeing, overeating, and obsessive thoughts about food are often used to deal with emotions, fears, and past traumas. The first step in recovery is to learn to interrupt these behaviors while at the same time not making them the focus of all your efforts.

Why is it necessary to stop doing these things? If you're not satisfied with your body, doesn't it make sense to put yourself on a diet? If you don't trust yourself to eat healthily, doesn't it make sense to be strict in how you think about food? The fact is, these strategies aren't effective because they don't address the deeper issues. For instance, the reason diets don't work is because they focus solely on the level of superficial behaviors. People are made to believe that if they just lose weight, their lives will change, their stress will go away, and they will somehow magically be comfortable around food when the diet ends. If you're reading this book, you have probably admitted to yourself on some level that dieting only makes things worse. For food addiction, abstinence means no longer practicing the behaviors associated with your eating addiction—such as eating impulsively, obsessing about food, restricting, and all the other behaviors that are part of your specific form of food or eating addiction. Your food addiction behaviors serve as a distraction from dealing with underlying issues in your life and allow you to stay in denial about other issues that you are not addressing.

Many definitions of recovery from food addiction require abstinence. Some definitions of abstinence put most of the spotlight on which foods to avoid (flour and sugar, for example, in the case of Food Addicts in Recovery Anonymous). Abstinence that requires restricting may, for some people, be very difficult to maintain and may also set you up for bingeing. If you feel that avoiding sugar and flour is best for you personally, you should definitely follow this path. For many people the 12 Steps and the fellowship of Alcoholics Anonymous, Overeaters Anonymous, and other Anonymous groups are very helpful and supportive. What is most important is that you weigh whatever you're being told against what you know works best for you. Sometimes it's hard to know for sure what does work for you, so it may require a period of being curious and of experimentation. If you stay mindful during such a period and are aware of how your behaviors affect you physically, mentally, and spiritually, you can't go wrong. (You will have a chance to write your own definition of abstinence in the exercise below.)

You may be convinced that you have to "demonize" certain foods in order to keep yourself from eating them. Or you may have convinced yourself that the only way to stop your behaviors is to try even more extreme diets, only to regain the weight you've lost and usually more. But it's deeply painful to be so hard on yourself. By thinking about Lisa's story, it may be easier for you to see how much pain your own behaviors are causing you. Not only does her secretive bingeing cause her a great deal of distress, but she also worries incessantly that her behaviors will be passed down to her daughter.

The first step to any change is becoming more aware of your behaviors. In order to develop this awareness in a way that doesn't create more shame or guilt, it is important to create a sense that this work is sacred. This will help you give yourself permission to avoid self-hatred or self-abuse about whatever you learn during this time. Let's start with creating a sacred space.

EXERCISE:
Creating Your Personal Sacred Space

Start by finding a comfortable place in your home where you are not likely to be disturbed. Quiet your mind by focusing on a memory of something that made you feel nurtured and cared about in the past. Perhaps it is something from childhood. Or maybe it's a memory of falling in love with your current partner or spouse. Or it may be a casual encounter with a beloved aunt or grandparent.

As you bring up this memory, think of any smells that you can recall. Think of any colors that were present. Remember what time of year it was. Recall the sounds that were part of the experience—for example, wind chimes that rang on the porch or music in the background.

Now focus all your attention on your heartbeat and see if you can remember how your heart felt during the experience. You may have felt your heart was full, or felt a sense of pure safety and connection, and this made your heart feel gentle and relaxed in your chest.

Continue for as long as you want to remember this wonderful, nurturing time. If for any reason negative thoughts distract you, see if you can gently return yourself to this memory.

You may not be able to think of such a memory. If this is the case for any reason, you can instead use an inspirational reading or listen to music that brings you joy and peace.

Then, when you feel ready, answer the questions below.

1. What is most sacred in your life? (For Lisa, her relationship with her daughter was the most sacred thing in her life.)

_____

_____

_____

2. How do you nurture and care for this most sacred thing in your life? (In Lisa's words: *I spend time with my daughter. I give her my undivided attention. I let her know how I feel about her.*)

_____

_____

_____

To bring the exercise to a close, take three deep breaths, feeling your breath moving from the top of your scalp, through your heart, and filling the rest of your body all the way to the tips of your fingers and toes. You can bring yourself back to this sacred space any time you need to.

_____

To let go of the superficial behaviors that are no longer serving you, you must first become aware of them. That will be the focus of the next exercise. It's important to be kind to yourself as you work to develop this awareness. If you find yourself becoming negative or self-judgmental, remind yourself that you have created a sacred space in which self-judgment is no more appropriate for you than it would be to judge the most sacred thing in your life. If you would nurture whatever or whomever is sacred to you, then see if you can extend the same sense of nurturing and acceptance toward yourself. It may be difficult at first, but you can keep yourself out of the negative zone by taking two or three deep breaths and recalling a time when you felt truly cared for, or reminding yourself of how you treat and care for what you hold sacred. Let's give it a try.

EXERCISE:
Observing Your Behaviors

Answer the questions below as if you were a fly on your own walls. Don't judge; only report on what is happening. If you get trapped in negativity, please use the techniques listed above or start from the beginning of the previous exercise to re-create (as many times as you need to) your sacred space.

1. What superficial behaviors have you engaged in around food and eating? This list is a description of what your personal eating addiction consists of. Put a check next to any of the things below that apply to you:

    ☐   Secretive eating

    ☐   Being "out of control" with certain foods

    ☐   Impulsive eating

    ☐   Hoarding food to eat later

    ☐   Bingeing

    ☐   Not allowing myself to eat foods my body is craving

    ☐   Allowing myself to overeat foods my body is craving

    ☐   Using other substances or behaviors to control how much I eat (cigarettes, caffeine, workaholism, shopping, and so on)

    ☐   Obsessive thoughts about food

    ☐   Obsessive thoughts about my body

    ☐   Extreme diets

    ☐   Compulsive eating when I'm no longer hungry

    ☐   Other: _____

    _____

2. Are there any other things you do that you think might really be about numbing yourself or reducing pain or distress? List them below. (Examples: *compulsive exercise, eating only "healthy foods," excessive weighing.*)

_____

_____

_____

_____

3. In the area below, please write your own personal definition of abstinence. How will you know when you are successful in your recovery? (Example—Lisa's definition of abstinence: *I will eat three meals most days of the week and will no longer skip meals. I will not eat on impulse. I will no longer eat while distracted by the TV, work, social media, or phone calls. I will have regular sit-down meals with my daughter. I will be more aware of how the food I eat makes my body feel. I will practice accepting my body and appreciating its strength and resilience.*)

_____

_____

_____

_____

_____

_____

Good work! You have taken an important first step on the road to long-term recovery. Just like you, Lisa was able to become more aware of her behaviors and to begin to interrupt some of them. When she set her definition of abstinence, she was surprised to find it wasn't all about her weight or about being able to eat whatever she wanted when she wanted. Next, Lisa worked on learning how her behaviors were being driven by the emotions that she was numbing with food.

Level 2—Emerging from the Emotional Soup

Once you're aware of the addiction-like behaviors you have around food, it's time to recognize that these behaviors are being driven by emotions. Essentially, you are using food as a way to cope with feelings. In Lisa's story, her self-confidence and sense of being safe in the world and being able to keep her daughter safe were marred by her traumatic childhood experience. That experience made her feel the need to be on red alert all the time—especially to keep her daughter safe. Being on red alert is an overactivation of your stress response system. For Lisa, this was associated with anxiety, difficulty relaxing, and feelings of fear. These emotions are what drove her to binge on sweets. Eating sweets made her feel better, if only temporarily.

Perhaps you have had similar adverse experiences—either as a child or later in your life. Or maybe you have a very demanding and stressful job that constantly wears you down. Or you may be in an abusive or unfulfilling relationship. There are many ways your emotions can be triggered, leading you to gravitate toward food. In some ways, obsessive thoughts about food can serve—either consciously or unconsciously—as a distraction from emotions that you don't know how to deal with. In part 3 of this book, you'll learn effective, healthy ways to cope with these emotions. But first, you must raise your awareness of what you're feeling and learn how those feelings can cause emotional eating, stress eating, and obsessive thoughts about food. The exercises below will help you identify situations in your life that may be bringing up emotions that trigger your overeating.

EXERCISE:
Identifying the Situations and Emotions
Connected to Your Food Addiction

Think of your most recent food binge, or the most recent time you found yourself obsessing about food to the point that it became a distraction from other things you needed or wanted to get done. Describe it in the space below. (Example: *Lisa had an argument with her mother. After the argument, she drove to her favorite chicken wings place and binged until she felt sick to her stomach. She missed a meeting at work because she didn't notice the time, as her focus was completely taken over by her need to eat those chicken wings.*)

_____

_____

_____

_____

Now identify emotions that you were feeling at the time, or right before. You may have to think back to something that happened the day before that you kept worrying about. (Example: *Lisa was really angry at her mother. Their argument had left Lisa feeling belittled and powerless.*)

_____

_____

_____

_____

List other situations that have directly or indirectly led to bingeing or other addictive food behaviors. Here are some possible ones to get you started.

- ☐ Argument with spouse or significant other

- ☐ Worrying about children, pets, or family members

- ☐ Incident at work or conflict at work

- ☐ Financial stress

- ☐ Conflict in the family

- ☐ _____

- ☐ _____

- ☐ _____

- ☐ _____

Next, think of how you feel before eating your trigger foods (foods you tend to obsess about or eat during binge episodes) and while you're eating them. The idea is to determine what emotional value those foods have for you:

Trigger food: _____

- ☐ When I think about eating this food, I feel _____

- ☐ While I'm eating this food, I feel _____

Trigger food: _____

- ☐ When I think about eating this food, I feel _____

- ☐ While I'm eating this food, I feel _____

Trigger food: _____

☐   When I think about eating this food, I feel _____

☐   While I'm eating this food, I feel _____

Take a moment to review your answers to the questions above. What did you learn about the connection between your emotions and your behaviors? (Example: *Lisa said she didn't realize how angry she was until she looked back on the situation. She had felt like the craving to stop at the wing shop "just hit" her and she couldn't drive by. She realized that eating the chicken wings had temporarily helped her feel calmer.*)

_____

_____

_____

_____

_____

    I hope you are beginning to get a glimpse into the vicious cycle created by unconscious emotions that drive you to engage in behaviors that make you feel better for a short time period but often, much worse later. You may feel as if the craving for a certain food "comes out of nowhere." However, if you stop and track it back, you will often be able to identify an emotion that was cut short before it even came into your conscious awareness. I would encourage you to continue this exercise, perhaps in your journal, to gain as many insights as you can. If you journal on this issue for several weeks, your increased awareness will be a valuable tool in interrupting your behaviors.

    You can change your behaviors only if you allow yourself to feel more of your emotions. This idea may seem frightening to you—and for good reason. Your family may never have allowed you to express your feelings. Or you may have gotten in trouble for crying or getting angry in the past. The exercise that follows will help you identify your personal history with emotional expression.

EXERCISE:
Family Rules About Emotional Expression

In the space below, describe how emotions were treated in your family when you were growing up. Were there rules such as "Big boys don't cry"?

_____

_____

_____

_____

_____

How have your family rules affected how you express emotions now?

_____

_____

_____

_____

_____

The key to breaking the trigger/emotion cycle is to allow yourself to experience your emotions. The goal should not be to avoid emotions, because that only makes them persist or become bigger and scarier (Blackledge and Hayes 2001). On the other hand, if you are able to fully experience your emotions, they tend to pass through you without causing damage. In the exercise below, you can learn how to do just that.

EXERCISE:
Expressing Your Emotions

Answer the questions below to start exploring how to express your emotions without using food.

In the section below, write down how you usually experience and express each of the emotions, including how you might use food to deal with the emotion. (Example: *Getting angry reminds me of my mother's rages when I was growing up. When she got angry at me I always felt diminished somehow. I felt that no matter how many times she said she loved me, her anger showed me that her love was conditional.*)

What does "get angry" mean to you?

_____

_____

When you get angry at someone or when someone gets angry at you, how does this feel?

_____

_____

What's your worst fear about what would happen if you got really angry?

_____

_____

What things do you do to avoid this emotion?

_____

_____

How have these avoidance strategies worked for you in the past?

_____

_____

Imagine now how it feels for you to be able to express your anger from a place of wanting to be true to your values. Describe what that would feel like:

_____

_____

_____

You can think of your emotions and thoughts associated with these emotions like a beach ball. If you try to hold the ball underwater, it will continually pop up in your face. What if you were able to allow the ball to just float around you without having to interact with it? Once you identify the meaning that these emotions have for you and become more aware of what your true value is, you can begin to see the emotions and the thoughts that go with them like a beach ball. How long do you want to try to hold it underwater? Whenever you actually feel an emotion, you're allowing that emotion—that beach ball—to exist, and it will eventually become less of a problem in your life as a result. If anger is not your most feared or unpleasant emotion, do the same exercise above with fear, shame, guilt, embarrassment, anxiety, or another emotion.

At times, you will probably need to remind yourself that it is normal to feel emotions and that it only feels abnormal because of the reasons you've listed above. Be gentle with your emotional self—it may be a very young part of yourself who was hurt or shut down. You need to allow that part of yourself time to heal. There's nothing to do other than to stay aware of the feelings and allow them to be there, rather than shutting them down immediately. If you are in a public place, or it isn't appropriate to express your emotions openly, at least acknowledge the emotion and see if you can make time and space later in your day to bring that feeling to the surface again and allow it to be expressed.

Another powerful way to access your emotion is through body sensations. This is what you'll learn about next.

Level 3—Embracing the Wisdom of Body Sensations

If, like Lisa, you've struggled with food and weight issues most of your life, you may have come to see your body as something separate from you and from your mind. Perhaps you respect your thoughts but don't respect the sensations in your body. You may feel your body is not your ally, but a recalcitrant and stubborn enemy that you're trying to beat in the game of weight loss. You may feel embarrassed by your body or feel your body is always throwing you a curve ball with random food cravings and desires, strange sensations that you don't understand and even stranger needs that may baffle you.

I won't try to convince you with logic that you should treat your body better, as that doesn't usually work. Instead, I'll offer some exercises to help you begin to understand how relevant body awareness and body respect are to your long-term recovery. By reclaiming a connection with your body and learning your body's language, you will be able to use your body's wisdom, which far surpasses anything your mind tells you, to help you heal. The mind and its constant barrage of thoughts, opinions, and judgments are where your food addiction lives. The body is where the healing happens.

EXERCISE:
Listening to Your Body's Wisdom

Let's start by understanding what kind of relationship you currently have with your body. Answer the questions below, while reminding yourself of the sacredness of the journey you are taking.

1. List below as many comments you've made about your body as you can remember. I've listed a few to get you started.

    ☐   *I can't remember the last time I could see my feet while standing.*

    ☐   *If I get any fatter/flabbier/uglier, no one will ever want to be with me.*

    ☐   *My legs are like tree stumps. I hate them.*

    ☐   _____

    ☐   _____

    ☐   _____

    ☐   _____

    ☐   _____

    ☐   _____

2. Now go back and reread the comments and imagine sitting in a coffee shop and overhearing a stranger say the exact same things about her body.

    a. What impressions would you have?

    _____

    _____

    _____

b.   What emotions would come up for you?

_____

_____

_____

3. What does your body represent to you? (For example, Lisa writes: *My body repre-sents all my failures. I feel like I can be great at my career and a good wife and mother, but my inability to control my body makes all that seem less meaningful.*)

_____

_____

_____

4. What do you think your body expresses about you? (For example, Lisa writes: *I feel like my body portrays me as someone who is weak.*)

_____

_____

_____

Next, think about how your body has served you in a beneficial or positive way throughout your life, and what kind of relationship you'd like to develop with your body.

5. What has your body done for you? How has your body helped you in life? (For example, Lisa writes: *My body delivered a beautiful baby girl. My body is strong. My body has survived trauma.*)

_____

_____

_____

6. If you could change your relationship with your body, what would you like to be different? (For example, Lisa writes: *I'd like to be able to look at myself in the mirror and not hate my body. I'd like to feel more comfortable in my skin.*)

    _____

    _____

    _____

7. What steps can you take right now to begin to shift your unhealthy relationship with your body to one that is more satisfying? (For example, Lisa writes: *Maybe if I start at least paying attention to the negative things I say about myself and then interrupt those negative thoughts at least part of the time, that would help.*)

    _____

    _____

    _____

    _____

Developing a new relationship with your body is not very different from changing patterns in a relationship with a friend or family member. If you grew up with siblings, you may have struggled with one or more of them at some point in your life. Or perhaps you had problems with someone in school or at work and over time you were able to work things out. In the same way, you can develop a better relationship with your body. Use the exercise below to explore this possibility further.

EXERCISE:
Rebuilding Your Relationship with Your Body

1. Think of any relationship you've had, or still have, that has taken some work in order to overcome differences or misunderstandings. Describe below what the challenges were in the relationship.

_____

_____

_____

2. Ask yourself what made you stick it out with this person rather than ending the relationship. Was it that you two had a long history? Did this person stick with you through troubled times?

_____

_____

_____

3. Now list specific skills you used and actions you took that worked to improve the relationship:

_____

_____

_____

4. Finally, explain how you can use similar skills and actions to rebuild your relationship with your body:

_____

_____

_____

Remember that every relationship needs time and space to grow. Don't put expectations on yourself that this will happen overnight. Try to work on it a little at a time, and always give yourself lots of positive feedback for even the smallest bit of progress. Before you know it, things will have changed for the better!

Level 4—Creating New Core Beliefs

A core belief is the lens through which we see ourselves, other people, and the world. Core beliefs are usually formed when we are young. They can also be formed in adulthood, when we've experienced a traumatic event or an emotionally distressful time. Core beliefs usually have to do with primal needs, such as the need for safety, attention, love, and approval. For Lisa, one of her core beliefs is that she is not safe. This belief was formed during her childhood trauma. Core beliefs usually serve a purpose when they are formed, but often they become problems for us later in life. For Lisa, for example, the belief that she is not safe may make it very difficult for her to be in an intimate relationship.

Once you form a core belief, you probably won't be consciously aware of it, but it will be one of the driving forces for your behaviors—not just behaviors relating to food, but to many other aspects of your life. For example, having a core belief that she was not safe made Lisa feel she had to be constantly vigilant. Constant vigilance is very stressful and makes it difficult to trust people. That could affect her ability to form relationships. It definitely would affect her eating behaviors, making her feel the need to closely monitor and control her choices about food (and perhaps her daughter's choices as well). This tendency could eventually harm Lisa's relationship with her daughter because her daughter may feel her mother is too controlling, not realizing why. Acting from a core belief that no longer supports you is like thinking you're sending out a certain message but having that message come across in a totally different way. For example, Lisa may want to have a relationship but her core belief (that protected her in childhood) will keep her from allowing herself to get close. So other people may perceive her as being aloof, when in fact that's not who she really is.

So it's important to understand what your core beliefs are and how they are operating in your life. In the exercise below, see if you can identify at least one core belief. You'll know when you've found a core belief because you will be able to see how the belief affects many areas of your life. You may also experience a physical sense of resonance, a feeling of *Yes, that's right!* Even if you think you know about one or more of your core beliefs, I invite you to do the exercise and see what else you can uncover. As you know, one of Lisa's core beliefs is that she's not safe. But there are others as well.

EXERCISE:
Finding Your Core Belief

Think of a situation that you are struggling with. It can be something that happened quite a while ago or more recently, but it should be a situation that you still feel emotional about—something that bothers you all over again whenever you think about it. Describe the situation below, including your emotions, thoughts, judgments, and opinions. (For example, Lisa writes: *My sister found out I was on a popular diet and she got very upset with me. She told me I was setting the wrong example for my daughter. She said that by now I should know that diets don't work and that with such a restrictive diet I would end up bingeing and gaining all my weight back. I felt angry and shamed. Who is she to tell me how to run my life and what's good for my daughter? I also felt afraid, because I think a part of me knew she was right. I felt that she has no idea how desperate I feel sometimes to lose weight because she doesn't have a weight problem. This happened a year ago and I still can't stop thinking about it. I can hardly look my sister in the face I get so mad at her.*)

_____

_____

_____

_____

_____

_____

_____

What behaviors did you engage in after the situation occurred? What do you do whenever you think about it and get upset all over again? (Example: *At first, I wanted to just show her that she was wrong, so I stayed on my diet and kept most of the weight off, but gradually it came back again as I went back to my old ways of bingeing on sweets. Sometimes when I think about it, I will eat a whole gallon of ice cream by myself.*)

_____

_____

_____

_____

_____

Now ask yourself what judgments you have about yourself when you think of this situation. What is the little voice in the back of your mind saying, late at night when you rehash the situation? (For example, Lisa writes: *If I weren't so weak, then I would have been able to stay on the diet and prove my sister wrong.*)

_____

_____

_____

_____

_____

Rewrite the statement you made above in the form of "I am _____," and you'll have your core belief—or at least a part of it. You may have a physical sensation that confirms that this is a core belief for you.

See if your statement fits the criteria of showing up in many other areas of your life. (Example: *For Lisa, the core belief of "I am weak" at first was hard to identify in other areas of her life because she was so good at covering it up. With deeper thought, she realized that she felt weak whenever she gave in in an argument with her husband or her boss. She felt weak when she wasn't able to stand up to her mother, who constantly harassed her about her weight.*) List as many examples as you can of how this core belief shows up in other areas of your life:

_____

_____

_____

_____

If you've had any trouble coming up with your core belief, choose another situation that is still bothering you and that has some emotional associations. Answer the following questions:

What do you believe it means about you that this situation happened?

_____

_____

_____

If you're still having trouble, imagine if this situation had happened to someone else—perhaps a friend or even a stranger. Be sure to let go of your thoughts about judging yourself or a "friend," and just look for the truth of what your friend might feel. See if you can dig deeper and find the nugget of truth—how your friend might really feel in her darkest moments when she thinks or "knows" that she should have done something differently. What judgment would your friend have about herself because of this situation?

_____

_____

_____

Now rewrite that judgment so it's about you.

_____

_____

If you find you are not able to identify a core belief, it's all right. You may not be ready, and you can always come back to this section when you do feel ready. Please don't judge yourself or think you've failed in any way because you have not yet been able to identify a core belief that resonates with you. As you learned from Level 3, the body has its own innate wisdom and knows when the time is right to go deeper and when the time is not right. This is an opportunity to trust your body's wisdom.

If you have identified a core belief, ask yourself if this belief is still working for you.

This is not just a yes or no type of question. Some parts of your core belief may be important for you to hold on to. Take, for example, Lisa's core belief of not feeling safe. She can use the knowledge that not everyone is trustworthy to help her protect her daughter. For instance, she would be very wise in thoroughly checking out any sitter or school situation before entrusting her child to their care. But the part of her belief about being unsafe that would not serve her is being paralyzed with fear and never allowing her daughter to take any risks—an approach that would definitely backfire and have negative effects for both her and her daughter. Her current core belief of feeling she is weak probably has no upside at all.

Are there any parts of your core belief that are still useful? What parts are not useful in any way? Are you ready to let go of the parts that aren't helpful anymore?

_____

_____

_____

_____

You will learn how to let go of your unhealthy core beliefs in part 3 of this book. For now, try keeping a journal (or a spreadsheet, if you prefer) to raise your awareness. Notice the ways in which your core belief is reflected in your life. Does it show up in relationships? How about at work? Is your core belief consciously or unconsciously in mind when you make decisions? This is information that will help you when the time comes to work further on your core beliefs.

Level 5—Finding Soul Satisfaction

When you have a food or eating addiction and have obsessive thoughts and uncomfortable behaviors about food, the suffering you experience is related to a difference between what your cravings and emotions are telling you to do and what you feel in your soul is authentic or true for you. Recovery from food addiction is very much about satisfying the true needs of your soul. People find soul satisfaction through a host of practices: meditation, being in nature, going to 12-Step meetings, or being part of any group that gives them positive, uplifting input. These practices can lift your spirits, give you a sense of awe, or simply make you feel good. This will be discussed in more detail near the end of the book. For now, the next exercise will help you begin to identify the practices that are working for you already, and others you may want to adopt to find soul satisfaction. Remember that these activities can be considered "natural positive reinforcers" that will help your brain make more dopamine and reduce the risks posed by RDS, as discussed previously.

EXERCISE:
Finding Soul Satisfaction

In the spaces below, make a list of practices you already have in place that lift your spirit, create awe, or make you feel happier. (I've listed some common ones to get you started.)

☐ Attending church regularly

☐ Spending time in nature

☐ Belonging to a supportive group of like-minded people who uplift me

☐ Praying regularly

☐ Meditating regularly

☐ Working with a sponsor

☐ Practicing yoga or qigong

☐ Engaging in breathing exercises

☐ Gardening

☐ Painting

☐ Volunteering

☐ _____

☐ _____

☐ _____

☐ _____

☐ _____

Take a moment to remind yourself of how to create a sense of sacred space by taking three deep breaths, recalling a memory of true caring, or reminding yourself of how you treat and care for what you hold sacred. Once you feel you are in that sacred space, answer the questions below.

If I were to eat to satisfy my soul, I would

_____

_____

If I were to use my emotions to satisfy my soul, I would

_____

_____

If I were to use my body to satisfy my soul, I would

_____

_____

If my core beliefs were to serve the purpose of satisfying my soul, they would include

_____

_____

If I were to put more of my focus on developing soul satisfaction, I would

_____

_____

_____

As natural positive reinforcers, any activity that gives pleasure—if not abused—will help heal the brain. This should be a priority in your healing journey. Take what you've discovered above and make a commitment to setting an intention to focus on developing at least one natural positive reinforcer in your life. You can state your commitment below. (Examples: I will explore how I can shift my relationship with my body (to satisfy my soul) by signing up for a yoga class at the YWCA. Or: I will go to Food Addicts in Recovery Anonymous at least once a week.) Write a statement of your commitment here:

_____

_____

Remember that healing the brain is an important part of healing the body and mind. As you discover other activities (natural positive reinforcers) that bring you pleasure and reward, you may find yourself relying less on food to fill that role. Look for classes you can take. Consider beginning an activity with a friend or family member. Journal about your responses to these activities. (You can access a guided imagery meditation exercise, "Journey of Discovery," at http://www.newharbinger.com/32097 that will help you use the tools in this chapter.) Most of all, remember to create space and time in your life to make the desired changes from a place of soul satisfaction, rather than feeling you need to do something for superficial reasons or feeling compelled to do something.

Shifting from the Quick Fix to the Long-Term Solution

This chapter is one step in helping you understand how to shift your thinking and your actions away from the quick fix of dieting, bingeing, and all the other behaviors that have brought you so much suffering, toward a more life-affirming way to live. What does it mean to make this shift?

Most people with food and body image issues hold on to the belief that the only thing keeping them from being fat or fatter is having to whip themselves in shape periodically, or getting mad at themselves when they "make a mistake." The negative self-talk and body hatred that go along with the diet mentality do not address in any way the underlying reason for your obsession with food. Remember that food addiction has its basis in personality traits such as impulsivity and compulsivity, trauma and abuse from childhood, or adverse early life experiences—all of which have created RDS, a genetic issue. There is no amount of whipping yourself into shape that will change your genes, remove trauma, or erase childhood neglect. So we need to redefine food addiction as not being just about losing weight.

In 2015, the American Society of Addiction Medicine changed its definition of addiction to state that "addiction is a chronic, relapsing brain disease..." (NIDA 2015). Food addiction is no different. It is chronic. It is caused by changes in the brain that affect the way you see and feel about food and your response to foods that are highly palatable. If you can accept the chronic nature of food addiction, you will understand that it is a long-term issue. It won't be fixed by any diet. Now, add into this that food addiction is a brain disease caused by the personality issues of impulsivity and compulsivity—part of RDS, which is partly a genetic problem—and you may be able to understand more deeply that you have to look for long-term solutions and you have to work at this over time.

This reality may seem discouraging until you think about how much time and energy you've already put into trying to get rid of your food addiction. What if you could spend time doing what really works—changing your lifestyle, learning about how to deal with RDS, and healing adverse childhood experiences and attachment disorders? What if you could focus on these very real issues, and with each action you take, with the time you invest, see significant long-lasting change? Would that be worth it for you? If so, keep reading.

Wrap-up

If you've been able to complete the exercises in this chapter, congratulations! If you have not fully completed them, don't be hard on yourself. Baby steps always beat no steps. The journey you are taking is sacred. It is one in which you will learn a lot about yourself from an informational point of view. But education rarely changes behavior, emotions, body image, or core beliefs. What will help you move through the Five Levels—besides time—is delving into each process, each exercise, with honesty and with an open heart. If you can allow yourself to be the observer without being the judge, your suffering will gradually be replaced with self-confidence and, more importantly, self-love.

CHAPTER 5

Understanding Your Body

Jonathan would be the first to tell you that he "lives to eat." He was overweight as a child, and as an adult his weight has gone over 300 pounds. He was thirty-five when he first came to my office and complained of a lot of symptoms that he thought might be related to his weight. He was experiencing severe joint pains that interfered with his ability to walk even short distances. He also reported frequent stomach upsets related to his food binges. Jonathan had a history of frequent sinus infections, seasonal allergies, depression, and anxiety. His doctor told him that his blood sugar was high and that he was prediabetic, which was very frightening because his mother had died from complications of diabetes. His job was stressful, he often felt overwhelmed at work, and his stress was contributing to his overeating. Jonathan had been on numerous fad diets but had never been able to maintain his weight at anything close to what his doctor told him was a "healthy weight." He was frustrated and demoralized by his inability to "fix the weight problem."

Because of Jonathan's difficulty losing weight and keeping it off, I wanted to find out whether he had any food sensitivities. He was tested and came back positive for moderate-to-severe gluten sensitivity. He was also sensitive to romaine lettuce and MSG (a flavor enhancer commonly used in Asian cuisine). Interestingly, Jonathan said the only kind of salads he would eat were made with romaine lettuce, and he ate out a lot at Asian restaurants. When he eliminated the foods he was sensitive to, his energy level increased and his joint pain decreased. He was able to continue enjoying Asian food by finding restaurants that were MSG-free. After six months, he had not had even one sinus infection and had lost thirty pounds without dieting.

Other testing showed that Jonathan had high levels of inflammation in the body and that his cortisol levels were reversed (higher in the evening than in the morning). This made it hard for him to go to sleep. I discussed with him how lack of sleep could also contribute to weight gain and explained that inflammation is the underlying cause of many chronic diseases—including diabetes. We added omega-3 fatty acids to his diet to help reduce inflammation, reduced his intake of foods that cause inflammation when consumed at high levels (such as animal products and processed foods), and increased his intake of fruits and vegetables. He responded well to improvements in his sleep habits and using a supplement containing melatonin and valerian to help him sleep better. He felt less overwhelmed and more able to handle stressful events in his life. Over the next year, his weight went down and he was able to be more active. Repeat testing showed that his blood sugar had normalized. He no longer had joint pain and he still had not had another sinus infection. He felt better about himself and even more committed to continue improving his health.

In chapter 4, you learned about the Five Levels of Healing from food addiction. As you can see with Jonathan's story, it's important not to neglect your physical health while you're learning to improve your emotional health. In this chapter, you will learn more about your body and how to respect it by caring for your physical health.

Understanding Your Body

To transform your relationship with food from one of fear, shame, and guilt, you must understand the ways in which food and your body interact.

The body communicates with you by giving you messages about its experiences. The body speaks through emotions, physical symptoms, and body sensations. Think of times when you've been in an uncomfortable situation and you had butterflies in your stomach, or the hair on the back of your neck stood up. Think of times when you've binged and your body has felt overfull or sluggish, or you had fatigue or headaches. All of these symptoms are messages from your body, giving you important feedback.

If you feel you're not getting these messages, it may be that you're not paying attention when your body speaks to you. It may be that you notice the symptoms or experiences, but you don't recognize them as messages. In this chapter, you'll learn how to listen to your body by understanding the body's innate functioning.

This is not a chapter about good foods or bad foods. This is a chapter about having a tool kit that will enable you to understand how your body works and why it does what it does. You'll learn about the impact of food sensitivities and how your body might communicate an aversion to certain foods. You'll learn about the importance of a healthy digestive system. You'll learn about hormones and their effects on food addiction. You'll also learn about how your brain, your metabolic system, and your immune system all talk to each other to keep you healthy, and how they let you know when they are out of balance. This information is offered to you as a way to nourish your body for good health, as opposed to eating certain foods to feed your emotions, to lose weight, or because of your food obsessions. Understanding your body will enable you to use the wise messages your body sends you to determine how best to change your relationship with food and your body.

If you find that any of the information in this chapter makes you feel as if you're being restricted from eating something you want or makes you think, *Why can't I just eat like everyone else?* you may want to seek more support in going through this process. Support is available through 12-Step groups for food addiction, from nutritionists or dieticians, and from health care providers. It's difficult to change patterns of a lifetime, so don't be surprised if you need support. Food addiction—like other addictions—can make you feel powerless in the face of foods you crave or obsess about. Listening to your body and seeking support are how you get through this journey to healing. Let's start this process by discussing a common issue among people who struggle with eating issues: food sensitivities.

Food Sensitivities

A food sensitivity or food intolerance is an adverse reaction to a specific food or food ingredient. It is not the same as a food *allergy*, which is associated with a specific immune system response that causes facial swelling, difficulty breathing, and digestive complaints and can sometimes be life-threatening (anaphylaxis). You are probably familiar with some of the common food allergies, such as allergies to peanuts, shellfish, other nuts, milk, and some kinds of fruit or spices.

Food sensitivities, as opposed to food allergies, often go undiagnosed. Food sensitivities can involve milder immune system reactions and can result in inflammation in the gut, leading to what is known as *leaky gut syndrome*, which will be discussed later in this chapter. While food *allergies* cause a reaction within thirty minutes, food sensitivities have a delayed reaction, so symptoms may not occur for up to seventy-two hours after you eat the food you're sensitive to. Food sensitivities not only affect you physically; they can also affect mood and behavior, causing depression or anxiety. It is estimated that food sensitivities affect 20 percent of the population (Nelson and Ogden 2008).

Potentially Problematic Foods

The foods that most commonly cause symptoms are eggs, wheat and other gluten-containing foods, corn, cow's milk, and some food additives (artificial coloring, sulphites, nitrates, MSG, and others) (Philpott and Kalita 2000). Let's look at some of the bigger offenders.

GLUTEN

If you have recurrent stomach issues or other mysterious symptoms that doctors have not been able to help you with, you may have been told that you should try a gluten-free diet. And you're not alone. Gluten is the name given to the proteins found in wheat. About one-third of adults in the United States report trying to decrease gluten in their diets, and more than 200 million restaurant visits per year include a request for a gluten-free menu item (NPD Group 2013). Over the past ten years there has been an explosion in the number of gluten-free products available in the marketplace, amounting to over $4.3 billion in sales.

It's unclear why there is such an increase in gluten-related disorders. It may be because of a higher gluten content in most modern wheat products, the sheer number of food products that contain gluten, or the high consumption of processed foods, many of which contain gluten. (Sapone et al. 2012). Gluten is found in too many foods to list here, but you can easily find this information on websites such as http://www.celiac.nih.gov (NIDDK, 2016).

Gluten sensitivity is not an allergic reaction to wheat, nor is it an autoimmune disorder like celiac disease, which affects people who are genetically predisposed. Celiac disease affects the small intestine, causing pain in the digestive tract, chronic constipation and diarrhea, anemia, fatigue, weight loss, malabsorption, and failure to thrive (in children). The disease is diagnosed with a blood test or intestinal biopsy. It runs in families, and people with a parent or sibling with celiac disease are at higher risk. It is important to rule out celiac disease because it is associated with an increased risk for other serious health problems, such as type 1 diabetes, multiple sclerosis, and intestinal cancers, to name a few.

If you have gluten sensitivity, your symptoms may be similar to those associated with celiac disease but with more symptoms outside of the digestive system. Common symptoms of gluten sensitivity include gas, abdominal pain, skin rash, foggy mind, depression, bloating, headaches, behavioral changes, bone or joint pain, fatigue, and unexpected weight gain. Like Jonathan, you may find that cutting gluten-containing foods out of your diet will make you feel better, and may also decrease your cravings.

DAIRY PRODUCTS

As with gluten, there is a difference between an *allergy* to dairy products and a sensitivity or intolerance. Cow's milk allergy is the most common food allergy in infants and young children. About 2.5 percent of children under the age of three are allergic to milk (Nadeau 2011). Most of these children will eventually outgrow their milk allergy. For adults who have difficulty with dairy, the more likely issues are sensitivity and intolerance. If you have dairy sensitivity, you could be sensitive to either casein or whey, or you could be lactose intolerant.

Dairy sensitivity (as opposed to lactose intolerance) involves an activation of the immune system, causing an inflammatory reaction. If you have dairy sensitivity, your symptoms may be mild to moderate or can result in true life-threatening reactions.

If you are lactose intolerant, you will have difficulty digesting the sugar in milk (lactose) because you are lacking the enzyme to break down that sugar. If you have lactose intolerance, your symptoms will be primarily digestive, with gas, bloating, diarrhea, and abdominal cramping. You should have no trouble digesting yogurt or hard cheeses, which are low in lactose and well tolerated by many people with lactose intolerance (Rozenberg et al. 2016).

Sometimes lactose intolerance can be part of a wider intolerance to foods with FODMAP carbohydrates (fermentable oligosaccharides, disaccharides, and monosaccharides and polyols).

Lactose intolerance is a factor in half of those with irritable bowel syndrome, and requires not just the elimination of lactose-containing foods, but also some fruits, vegetables, beans, nuts, and grains, as well as high-fructose corn syrup and artificial sweeteners (Deng et al. 2015). If elimination of dairy does not relieve your gastrointestinal symptoms, you might consider a FODMAP-free diet under the supervision of a nutritionist.

Food Sensitivities and Food Addiction

About one-half of people with FS report having cravings for the very foods they are sensitive to. Researchers think that this is due to the production of natural endorphins in the brain. When the endorphins wear off, you may crave the food that provided these feel-good chemicals (Crawford and Cadogan 2008). Incomplete digestion of both gluten and dairy protein stimulates the production of opioid-like substances (casomorphins and gluteomorphins) that contribute to an addictive sensation and result in food cravings. Both gluteomorphins and casomorphins have been found in the urine of people with depression, schizophrenia, autism, and attention deficit disorder (Crawford and Cadogan 2008). Therefore, testing for food sensitivities (discussed later on in Medical Tests to Consider) can enable you to identify some of the underlying causes of food cravings.

If you have any of the symptoms listed in this chapter, you may want to consider getting tested for food sensitivities through your naturopathic, chiropractic, or integrative medicine health care provider.

In the section below, you will learn what you can do to get help for this problem. For further help, you can use the chart opposite to do a little personal detective work and track foods you eat and any symptoms that might be related to them.

EXERCISE:
Food and Symptoms Diary

In the chart opposite, list all foods you eat, along with drinks, snacks, medications, and supplements. List and date any symptoms you experience, including feelings of anxiety, depression, fatigue, and other symptoms you have noticed. You may be able to identify a pattern associated with eating certain foods. Just remember, your symptoms may occur as long as two to three days after eating a food you are sensitive to. (A downloadable version of this chart is available at http://www.newharbinger.com/32097.)

Date and time	Food eaten	Symptoms	How long did symptoms last?	Date and time of symptoms

Treatment of Food Sensitivities

If you think you may have a food sensitivity or intolerance, the first step is to determine whether you truly are sensitive to or intolerant of a food and, if so, *which* food or foods. There are two main ways to do this: medical testing or an elimination diet. In some cases, it makes sense to combine the two.

The food elimination diet (discussed below) is a good way to self-diagnose common food sensitivities if you prefer not to do testing.

ELIMINATION DIETS

The use of an elimination diet protocol can give you a clear idea of which foods are the cause of your symptoms. Typically, you would test yourself by eliminating from your diet the most common causes: dairy, eggs, peanuts, tree nuts, soy, and wheat. After three weeks, you reintroduce each food category one at a time, noticing any return of symptoms (or new symptoms you didn't notice before). For example, add in gluten-containing foods for one to two weeks and notice any symptoms. Then add in dairy foods. You might want to add in milk for one week, and then add cheese, as different proteins in milk (curds and whey) may affect you differently.

Any type of food restriction can trigger binge eating or food cravings. If you have any problems staying on the elimination diet, then it may be a better idea to do the blood test for food sensitivities. With the blood test, you will know exactly what you need to eliminate.

At the end of this chapter is a sample chart of foods to avoid and those that are safe to eat while you are on the elimination program. **Caution: if you develop an allergic reaction with swollen lips or throat, trouble breathing, or a severe rash, get medical assistance right away and do not proceed with the food challenge unless supervised by a physician.**

An elimination diet takes time and effort, but it will be worthwhile. Hopefully, as you read this chapter, you are starting to recognize that what you eat should not be looked at through the lens of what will make you lose weight. The foods you eat are much more important than that. What you eat can make the difference between feeling good or not, and being healthy or not. Understanding this is an important transition in your relationship with food and your recovery from food addiction.

Leaky Gut Syndrome

Although modern medicine has been slow to acknowledge the important role that gut function plays in disease, even in ancient times physicians were well aware of the connection between the gut and the brain. The father of modern psychiatry, French psychiatrist Philippe Pinel, said in 1807, "The primary seat of insanity generally is in the region of the stomach and intestines." Even before that, Hippocrates (460–370 BCE), the father of modern medicine, said: "All diseases begin in the gut!"

All throughout your intestinal tract are cells that form a lining in the intestinal wall, a barrier from the external environment. Leaky gut syndrome (also called intestinal permeability) results from damage to this lining, which allows bacteria, toxins, poorly digested proteins, and fats that are not normally absorbed to leak out of the intestines into the bloodstream. These products can trigger an immune system reaction that can cause abdominal and body-wide symptoms and inflammation. Inflammation is thought to be the underlying cause of most chronic medical conditions—heart disease, diabetes, obesity, and so on.

Researchers suggest that some people are more susceptible to changes in this barrier, and that these changes can be triggered by something from the environment, such as food sensitivities, stress, or toxins. Our modern lifestyle, including a western diet that promotes inflammation, is one of the causative factors. In studies in which animals are bred to be susceptible to diabetes, it has been shown that when they are given a normal diet, they will develop diabetes. When kept on a special anti-inflammatory diet, fewer of them develop diabetes. Interestingly, increased intestinal permeability is also present in humans with insulin-dependent diabetes (Arrieta et al. 2006). If you are overweight or obese, you are more likely to have an imbalance in gut bacteria (gut microbiome) and intestinal permeability (Bischoff 2011; Camilleri et al. 2012). One reason for this is that people with obesity are at higher risk for deficiencies in vitamins A and D—two vitamins that help protect the intestinal barrier (Lima et al. 2010; Sun 2010; Trasino et al. 2015).

Treatment of Leaky Gut Syndrome

To heal leaky gut syndrome, it is important to focus on reestablishing normal gut flora and healing and sealing the damaged gut lining. Healing the digestive system stops toxins in the gut from going to the brain, and removes or improves mental and physical symptoms. Once the gut is able to function normally, your food will be digested and absorbed properly, which is the key to overall physical and mental health (Holford 2003). If you are concerned about leaky gut syndrome or if you would like to find out whether there are imbalances in your gut bacteria, you can get tested through an integrative medicine physician or a naturopathic doctor.

Below are some suggestions you can use to help heal leaky gut syndrome. If you have any other serious physical or mental problems or are taking medications, you should consult with your health care provider before taking supplements.

1. Prebiotics—nondigestible carbohydrates (usually soluble food fibers) that act as food for probiotics. The best prebiotics are inulin and oligofructose. These two substances are found in chicory root, wild yams, other root vegetables, jicama, agave, whole grains, bananas, onions, garlic, honey, and artichokes. Prebiotics are also found in supplement form in health food stores. A good starting dosage of inulin or oligofructose is 4 grams daily. Consult your doctor about brand and dosage before taking.

2. Probiotics—live microorganisms that promote healthy bacteria in the gut, help reduce inflammation, and improve nutritional and immune status in the body. Use a product that contains a mix of different bacteria, including *Lactobacillus GG*, *Sacchromyces boulardii*, and *Bifidobacteria* (Crawford and Cadogan 2008). Consult your doctor about the brand and dose that is best for you.

3. Glutamine—an amino acid (building block of protein) that is important for helping boost immune function and removing ammonia (a waste product) from the body. Glutamine may also be necessary for normal brain function and digestion.

   Dose: Glutamine supplements (as L-glutamine)—500 mg–1000 mg daily. Glutamine is also available in most protein powders. Do not take with warm or hot beverages. Do not take if you have kidney or liver disease or a history of seizures. Do not take higher doses unless under the supervision of a physician.

4. Omega-3 fatty acids containing EPA and DHA to reduce inflammation in the body.

   Dose: 1000–3000 mg of combined EPA and DHA daily.

It is likely that Hippocrates was right. Recent research studies are supporting his view that gut health can affect both physical and mental disorders. In the case of food addiction, it's not surprising that cravings, bingeing, and obesity may begin with poor gut health caused by food sensitivities, overuse of antibiotics, trauma, stress, nonsteroidal anti-inflammatory drugs, cancer drugs and radiation, or excessive alcohol consumption.

Hormones and Food Addiction

Hormones are chemical messengers that work in complex, interrelated ways to control just about every process in your body, from appetite, food cravings, and metabolism to stress and emotions. Learning more about your hormones can go a long way in helping you understand how your body works and how to care for it. There are many hormones that relate to eating: ghrelin, made in your stomach, which stimulates appetite; leptin, made in the brain, which tamps down appetite; and neuropeptide Y, which makes you feel hungry—to name a few. Many of these hormones you have no control over, so this section will start by focusing on hormones that you may be able to exert some influence over in your desire to end your obsessive thoughts and behaviors relating to food. We'll also take a look at the relationship among hormones, emotional stress, and the immune system, and discuss how this triad relates to appetite, eating, and weight.

Insulin

Insulin is the hormone responsible for regulating blood sugar. It is also an important hormone when it comes to deciding whether the energy in the food you eat gets used up right away or, if not, is stored as fat. When food is stored as fat, the fatty tissue doesn't just remain dormant. Other hormones that affect appetite, cravings, and food intake are made directly by that fatty tissue.

Most of the food you eat is turned into glucose (sugar) in the body. Normally, the pancreas secretes enough insulin to clear glucose from the bloodstream. When glucose is too high on a consistent basis, or when the pancreas can no longer secrete enough insulin to clear the glucose, you may be diagnosed as prediabetic or diabetic. Some experts feel that regulation of blood sugar (whether or not you have diabetes) may be the most important nutritional change you can make (Maida et al. 2016).

Insulin levels are directly related to what you eat. Unfortunately, the standard American diet is a major cause of poorly regulated blood sugar. The best way to keep blood sugar balanced is to eat foods high in protein, avoid processed foods, and eat a balanced diet, including vegetables and healthy fats.

Balancing blood sugar and keeping insulin levels within normal ranges can be complicated. Here are some ways that blood sugar gets destabilized:

- Caffeinated drinks cause a release of sugar into the bloodstream.

- Stress—including job stressors, family conflict, loss, pain, allergies, and more—can also cause blood sugar to increase.

- Alcohol consumption interferes with the normal use of sugar in the body and causes insulin to spike. In reaction to the insulin spike, blood sugar may then drop too low and cause sugar cravings.

- Physical inactivity makes it hard for your body to use insulin effectively, leading to insulin resistance.

To improve your blood sugar stability, it is important to eat regularly throughout the day, include fruits and vegetables in your diet, and reduce your intake of foods that destabilize blood sugar. The exercise below will help you to do this.

EXERCISE:
Stabilizing Your Blood Sugar

In the exercise below, pick one or two changes in your eating pattern that you are willing to try to help stabilize your blood sugar:

☐ Add healthy fats to your diet. (Example: *Add avocado to your salad or use olive oil instead of corn oil.*)

☐ Take a five-minute walk every day.

☐ Find substitutes for sugary drinks and avoid artificial sweeteners.

☐ Eat a vegetable of your choice at least once daily.

☐ Add protein to your breakfast. (Example: *Eat one to two eggs, or add walnuts to your cereal or oatmeal.*)

☐ Add protein to your snacks. (Example: *Add peanut butter or almond butter to apple slices.*)

☐ Drink six to eight glasses of water daily.

Work your way through the list as you feel comfortable. Don't feel as if you need to change everything all at once. At every moment that you can take positive action, you strengthen your body's ability to do its job of balancing your blood sugar.

Thyroid Hormones

The thyroid gland is located at the base of your neck, above your collarbone. The thyroid essentially regulates your metabolism and body weight. Its other functions include regulation of menstrual cycles, body temperature, cholesterol levels, heart rate, and more. The thyroid gland can either underproduce thyroid hormone, causing weight gain and other symptoms, or overproduce, causing weight loss and other symptoms. Symptoms that may indicate a problem with your thyroid are fatigue; weakness; weight gain or difficulty losing weight; coarse, dry hair; hair loss; frequent muscle aches; constipation; and depression. If you have any of these symptoms, and particularly if you have a family member with a history of low thyroid (hypothyroidism), you should get tested by your health care provider.

Sex Hormones

Estrogen, progesterone, and testosterone are the sex hormones. These hormones have an impact on your appetite, weight, and food intake. Estrogen may help in regulating your appetite by stimulating the production of serotonin, which makes you feel full or satiated. Many women have changes in their appetite and food preferences around the time of their menstrual cycles that can be related to an imbalance between estrogen and progesterone, triggering food cravings. Testosterone affects weight and muscle mass. If you are female and are deficient in testosterone because of poor nutrition or perimenopause, you will not be able to build muscle as easily as someone with adequate testosterone. This deficiency can also affect your ability to burn calories and lose weight. The same can happen to men who have low testosterone levels that lead to a less muscular physique and a higher level of body fat. If you eat a very low-fat diet, you will not have adequate levels of the sex hormones that rely on intake of fat and cholesterol, the building blocks of all the sex hormones.

It can be difficult to tell if you have deficiencies in any of the sex hormones. Possible indicators include decrease in sex drive, weight gain, sleep problems, irregular menstrual cycles, fatigue, and depression. If you are concerned about possible deficiency in your sex hormones, your health care provider can do simple blood tests to determine whether your levels are normal, and can prescribe bioidentical hormone therapy or testosterone replacement if warranted.

Stress Hormones

Emotional stress has a number of direct and indirect effects on your eating, weight, and health. Stress influences your overall health because it affects a very important system in the body—the neuroendocrine immune (NEI) system, which includes the brain, metabolism, and the immune system. When one part of the NEI is out of balance, it can affect all three.

Emotions actually stimulate parts of the brain that affect the release of neurotransmitters (such as serotonin, dopamine, and norepinephrine) and also the production of certain hormones—some of which govern eating and weight. If you have a high level of emotional stress, you may experience anxiety, anger, fatigue, low mood, food cravings, weight gain, addiction, and difficulty sleeping. You may also have frequent colds or flu symptoms or recurrent infections, signaling that your immune system is not functioning properly. If your stress becomes chronic, the immune system produces inflammatory molecules called cytokines that increase inflammation in the body, causing further imbalances in the NEI system.

Stress can contribute to obesity by leading to "comfort" food eating or emotional overeating, lack of sleep that is associated with weight gain, impulsive behaviors, and overeating of highly palatable foods high in sugar, fat, and salt. Emotional stress leads to the activation of the body's stress system and the release of the stress hormones adrenaline, noradrenaline, and cortisol. Once your body's stress system is activated and you go into "fight-or-flight" mode, these stress hormones have their own negative effects on the body and can lead to the development of central obesity (apple figure), insulin resistance, and metabolic syndrome (characterized by high blood pressure, high cholesterol and triglycerides, and diabetes) (Pervanidou and Chrousos 2011).

If you have been under chronic emotional stress or you have experienced trauma in your life, it is likely that your cortisol levels are higher than normal. This can lead to disturbances in the immune system functions and contribute to the development of obesity, depression, and metabolic syndrome (Martinac et al. 2014). Later in this book, you will learn how to manage your response to stress to help minimize the release of these harmful hormones.

Medical Tests to Consider

Your body is not a machine. As you've learned in this chapter, it responds to your emotions, the stress in your life, whether you are active or sedentary, and the foods you eat. Once you understand how your body works, you will know that regular medical care is important. If you have one of the health conditions discussed in this chapter, it will be essential that you take good care of your body by identifying and treating the condition. Here is a list of tests that may be useful to bring with you to your next checkup.

Ask your health care provider whether any of these tests are recommended for you:

- [ ] Complete blood count. If you are female and have not gone through menopause yet, you can become anemic because of your monthly periods.

- [ ] C-reactive protein—a marker for overall body inflammation.

- [ ] Hormone levels. Estradiol, FSH, and free testosterone are the most commonly tested.

- [ ] Thyroid hormone testing. TSH tests screen for thyroid dysfunction. If abnormal, free T4 and other tests may be ordered.

- [ ] Fasting blood glucose—to determine if your blood sugar is high, which could indicate a risk for diabetes.

  - [ ] Hemoglobin $A1_C$. If your blood glucose is high, your doctor may want to determine whether it is chronically high or not.

Ask your integrative medicine or naturopathic doctor about:

- [ ] Intestinal permeability. This test may include information about leaky gut syndrome and about the state of your gut health (bacterial balance).

- [ ] Food sensitivities. Testing can identify specific foods and the level of sensitivity you have to these foods. You can then eliminate foods that may be causing intestinal permeability, food cravings, or inflammation.

- [ ] Hormone testing. Some providers believe the saliva test is more accurate than the blood test in giving an overall average of hormone levels over time.

- [ ] Stress index. This type of test usually measures the level of cortisol over a twenty-four-hour period and may also include other tests to check on the effects that stress is having on your body.

- [ ] Amino acid testing. This test may give you an estimate or a snapshot of the levels of neurotransmitters (serotonin, dopamine, and so on) in your brain and how they compare with what is thought to be normal. This may help your provider prescribe supplements or medication for depression, anxiety, or sleep issues.

Wrap-up

Physical health is the foundation of every other aspect of your life, including your mental and emotional well-being. As you've learned in this chapter, the food you eat directly affects the health of your body, and at the same time the various digestive and hormonal processes taking place within your body influence your appetite, cravings, and weight. We eat for many reasons. Some of those reasons have nothing to do with physical hunger or pleasure. One author put it this way: "Food literally speaks to your body and your body will answer back. Speak in a loving tone (eat 'real' food and actually 'understand' your body) and your body will respond in kind" (Crawford and Cadogen 2008). By coming to understand how your body works and learning to listen to your body's messages, you can cultivate a new relationship of care and respect for your body. This process will evolve over time as you become more aware of the wise messages your body is sending to you. In the next chapter, you'll learn more about helping your body break the hold food has on it.

Resources

1. To find a naturopathic doctor in your area, visit the website of the American Association of Naturopathic Physicians: http://www.naturopathic.org.

2. To find an integrative medicine doctor in your area:

    a. Arizona Center for Integrative Medicine (trains physicians in integrative medicine): http://www.integrativemedicine.arizona.edu.

    b. Academy of Integrative Health and Medicine (formerly the American Holistic Medical Association): http://www.aihm.org.

PROTEIN

Allowed: chicken, turkey, lamb, wild game, buffalo, elk, venison cold-water Fish: (halibut, herring, mackerel, salmon, sardines and tuna) beans, mushrooms and veggie burgers

Protein powder – hemp, pea, and rice protein with at least 7 grams per serving

Avoid: red meat, processed meats, eggs, and egg substitutes

STARCHES

Allowed: potatoes, rice, buckwheat, millet, quinoa, acorn squash, beets, parsnips, yams, plantains, and butternut squash

Avoid: gluten- and corn-containing pastas, breads, and chips

SWEETENERS

Allowed: brown rice syrup, fruit sweeteners

Avoid: brown sugar, honey, fructose, molasses, and corn syrup

DAIRY

Allowed: rice milk, hemp milk, coconut milk, flaxseed milk, and almond milk

Avoid: milk, cheese, ice cream, butter, cottage cheese, yogurt (dairy and soy), frozen yogurt, and whey

FATS / OILS

Allowed: cold/expeller pressed, unrefined, light-shielded canola, flax, olive, pumpkin, sesame, and walnut oils; avocados, olives, and salad dressing

Avoid: margarine, shortening, butter, and spreads

LEGUMES

Allowed: all legumes

Avoid: soy products (edamame, miso, soy sauce, tamari, soy milk, soy yogurt, textured vegetable protein, tofu, tempeh)

VEGETABLES

Allowed: all whole vegetables

Avoid: creamed or processed vegetables

NUTS / SEEDS

Allowed: almonds, cashews, pecans; flax, pumpkin, sesame, and sunflower seeds; and butters from allowed nuts and seeds

Avoid: peanuts, pistachios, and peanut butter

BEVERAGES

Allowed: fresh or unsweetened fruit/vegetable juices; herbal teas; filtered, spring, or sparkling water; and unsweetened coconut water

Avoid: Avoid: dairy, coffee, tea, alcohol, citrus drinks, and sodas

SOUPS

Allowed: any clear, vegetable-based soups

Avoid: canned or creamed soups

BREADS & CEREALS

Allowed: any made from rice, quinoa, amaranth, buckwheat, teff, millet, potato flour, or arrowroot

Avoid: all made from wheat, spelt, kamut, barley, rye, triticale, emmer, or farro

FRUITS

Allowed: most fruits

Avoid: strawberries and citrus

CHAPTER 6

Breaking Free from the Foods That Hold You Hostage

Christie is the single mother of one son and works in a legal office. She has been moderately overweight since her son was born. Her weight is only part of the problem. What bothers her most is her inability to stop bingeing on foods that people bring into the office or snacks that she buys and keeps at home for her son. She feels like a failure because she is completely unable to stop herself from eating these foods. She thinks about her favorite foods all the time. She always thinks she'll be able to stop after one small bowl of ice cream but inevitably she ends up eating the whole pint. She even hides ice cream from her son so she can have it all to herself. At work, she nibbles on foods brought in for holidays or birthdays when her coworkers are around. After everyone else has left, she finds herself coming back over and over again to get "small plates" until she realizes that she's eaten a lot more than she intended. After her out-of-control binge, she feels sluggish and her stomach is bloated and full of gas. She has had joint pains and recurrent headaches for the past year that she was told were due to her weight.

Christie finally realized that she was totally unable to stop her food obsessions and came to my office for help. Her food sensitivity testing showed that she was very intolerant of dairy products—the foods she was most likely to binge on. Christie at first embraced these results and stopped all dairy for two months. Her joint pain decreased and she didn't have any migraines during that period. Then, Christmas came and with it her favorite ice cream—peppermint crunch. She thought it wouldn't hurt to eat just one small bowl. Unfortunately, one bowl led to another and another. The next morning Christie woke up with severe joint pain and abdominal bloating. Using willpower to stay away from dairy hadn't worked. All her cravings had come back and she was having trouble learning how to deal with them. Christie needed help learning to accept a dairy-free lifestyle. She needed to work on detoxifying not just her body but also her mind. Over time, she was able to accept a dairy-free lifestyle and her health continued to improve—physical and emotionally.

In chapter 5, you learned more about underlying factors that contribute to your obsessions with food, including food sensitivities, stress, hormones, and intestinal permeability or leaky gut syndrome. Hopefully, this knowledge has started to shift your understanding about how your body works and the important role food plays in keeping you healthy. In this chapter, you will learn more about what to do when you can't stop yourself from eating foods that you obsess about.

Perhaps you've heard the term "detox" used to describe the first step in overcoming an addiction. In the case of food addiction, you need to detoxify both your body and your mind. Your body has likely suffered the toxic effects of foods it doesn't tolerate. Your food addiction may also have been made worse by toxins in your environment, through a process I'll explain below. And finally, when you struggle with food and eating, your mind is awash in toxic thoughts—that is, ways of thinking that keep you obsessed, hopeless, and feeling bad about yourself. Detoxifying both your mind and your body is the next step in breaking the hold food has on your life.

Detox for Your Body

One of the first ways you can begin to reduce your food obsessions and help your body stop craving these foods is to reduce as many causes of food cravings as you can. In the previous chapter, if you tried the elimination diet, you may have identified foods that affect your body in a negative way—causing cravings, physical symptoms, out-of-control eating, and weight gain. The first step is to treat your body kindly by choosing not to eat these foods. Another way of giving your body a clean slate to stop these unwanted cravings is through detoxification. In the first half of this chapter, we'll look more closely at detoxifying the body.

How Toxins Contribute to Food Addiction

Detoxification has a long tradition of being used as a way to cleanse or purify the body. Why should you be interested in this? If you have food addiction, it is likely that toxic chemicals in your environment have some impact on your cravings, on the types of foods you are craving, and on your impulsive and compulsive behaviors.

How might this be? Toxins affect the brain and nervous system, which control all of your behaviors, thoughts, emotional responses, and obsessions, including those associated with food. Exposure to toxins in the environment has been linked to hormonal disruptions, mood, and cognitive and neurological issues (Cummings et al. 2010; Grandjean et al. 2008; Soto and Sonnenschein 2010; Takser et al. 2005; Wuttke et al. 2010). Many toxins are stored in fatty tissues in the body and cause disruptions in the hormonal functions of fatty tissue, including having a role in cravings, inflammation in the body, energy, and brain function. Disruptions in these hormones have also been associated with relapse in women with drug addiction (Wilcox and Brizendine 2006).

Hormonal damage caused by environmental toxins has been associated not only with mood changes and sleep disturbance (Crinnion 2000) but also with changes in weight and appetite. Research has shown that if you have certain toxic chemicals in your body tissues, you are more likely to be overweight or obese (Baillie-Hamilton 2002). It's not only alternative medicine practitioners who are talking about this issue. The National Institutes of Health, the US Food and Drug Administration, and the Environmental Protection Agency have convened to discuss just this topic—how toxins cause obesity (Hyman 2010).

Every day, you are exposed to tens of thousands of pesticides, dyes, pigments, medicines, flavorings, perfumes, plastics, solvents, and other chemical agents. In the news, there are more studies than ever before showing that the level of toxins in our drinking water and in our soil is a problem. Toxins that you come in contact with are often stored in the body for extended periods of time—meaning that they can affect you long after you have been exposed. Symptoms of exposure to toxic chemicals are too numerous to list. The best resource for identifying toxins you may have been or are now being exposed to is the Environmental Working Group's website (http://www.ewg.org), which lists toxins in food, water, and cosmetics. In the next section, you will learn some specific steps to take to eliminate or reduce your exposure to toxins.

Detoxifying Your Body to Help with Food Addiction

You can help your body heal from food addiction through detoxification. Here are some ways to reduce the toxic burden that may be contributing to your food cravings and your weight (Hyman 2010).

1. To support your body's natural ability to get rid of toxins, include some of these foods in your meals: cabbage, broccoli, collards, kale, brussels sprouts, bok choy, arugula, mustard greens, and turnips.

2. Use the spices turmeric and curry in your cooking—they are known to help the liver rid the body of toxins.

3. Drink green tea, which increases glutathione—a strong antioxidant that helps the body repair itself and get rid of toxins.

4. Eat foods that contain sulfur: eggs, garlic, and onions. Sulfur is also important in the detoxification process.

5. Take supplements such as those listed below. (Consult your health care provider for information and advice about appropriate doses.)

   • N-acetyl cysteine—a supplement that increases glutathione.

   • Milk thistle—also increases glutathione.

   • Buffered vitamin C—helps keep the body's glutathione from being used up.

6. Eat organic foods when possible. Choose organic especially for the foods that are on the "dirty dozen" list (the Environmental Working Group's list of the produce that is the most contaminated with pesticides) (http://www.ewg.org).

7. Saunas and steam rooms have been used for generations as a tool for detoxification of heavy metals and fat-soluble toxins. If you have access to these therapies, give them a try.

By clearing your body of environmental toxins and foods you may be sensitive to, you give yourself the gift of a fresh start. In the next section, you will learn about releasing the hold that food has on your mind.

Detox for Your Mind

Shifting the ways of thinking that reinforce your obsession with food is also an important part of the process of transforming your food addiction. Food addiction involves an obsessive, compulsive, and impulsive relationship with food. Eating is so automatic that you may not realize how much your thoughts and emotions play into what you eat, how much you eat, and why you crave your food fixes. Because your response is so automatic, you may feel as if you will never be able to break the hold that food has on you.

In the next section, you will learn about how being more present and mindful about what you're doing can help you identify these patterns and reduce shame and guilt. Being mindful is like being a fly on the wall and having the emotional distance from your actions that allows you to see what's going on. A fly doesn't judge what it sees. When you interrupt the judgment, you can see more clearly why you do what you do, and this clarity will enable you to interrupt and change what is no longer working for you.

Mindful Awareness Is the Key

The only way to break the vicious cycle of cravings and binges and obsessive thoughts about food and your body is through awareness. You've probably heard the term "mindfulness" before, but perhaps you didn't realize how it applies to your situation. Being mindful means simply being present in the moment. How many times in your day do you think you are truly present? Are you present with your children? With your spouse or partner? Are you present at your job? Or are your thoughts always wandering, racing, and obsessing?

When you are not present in the moment, you may notice that your thoughts take on a life of their own. You may feel trapped in an automatic, vicious circle when you allow your thoughts and emotions to run the show. The alternative is mindfulness.

Mindfulness practices have great power to help you overcome food and body image issues. A review of multiple studies on mindfulness-based interventions was able to show a significant decrease in binge eating, emotional eating, and eating in response to environmental triggers (driving by a fast-food restaurant, for example) with the use of mindfulness strategies such as meditation, mindful eating, and others (O'Reilly et al. 2014). This training works by increasing awareness of the meanings behind cravings and learning to accept one's experience in the moment without judging it (Witkiewitz et al. 2013).

Eckhart Tolle may have said it best when he was interviewed on *The Oprah Winfrey Show*: "Being in touch with the body helps greatly because the body knows what it needs. Overeating happens because it is part of the ego's unconsciousness, which seeks to substitute for the sense of aliveness" (Davis, 2008). When food is substituted for a sense of aliveness or for soul satisfaction (part of the Five Levels discussed earlier in this book), it can never truly fill that need. You may feel a sense of discomfort, dissatisfaction, or letdown after a binge for this very reason: food isn't giving you what you truly need. By being more conscious of your thoughts and emotions, by being more attentive, the balance of power may shift in your relationship with food.

Cultivating Mindfulness

It may seem as if your experience of food addiction and all the behaviors, thoughts, cravings, and emotions associated with it overcome you and are automatic and unconscious. Being on autopilot may feel good in some ways, but when you "wake up" or become conscious or present again, you may be flooded with negative emotions and self-judgment about your behaviors. It only makes sense, then, that staying conscious by learning to stay in touch with your body and your thoughts and emotions will help you avoid those behaviors and the negative emotions that follow. It's all about where your attention is. When you are in the midst of a binge, your attention is on something outside yourself. While you may pay excessive attention to the appearance of your body, you may be completely unaware of the roles your body plays in your life that have nothing to do with your appearance.

STEP 1: WAKING UP

The first step is, therefore, to increase your awareness of and attention to each moment—with special emphasis on the moments that immediately precede your binges, cravings, or obsessive thoughts about food. In the exercise below, you will be able to identify those early moments so that you can be more aware of an action you *might* take before you find yourself in the middle of the behavior.

EXERCISE:
Waking Up

This exercise will walk you through a series of questions to analyze the thoughts, emotions, and sensations that go along with your out-of-control behaviors with food. When you have a deeper understanding of your triggers, you'll be in a better position to resist them.

1. List the behavior or action associated with your food addiction that causes you the most distress or suffering. Some examples are listed to help you get started, or you can write in your own in the space below:

   ☐ *What bothers me the most is when I feel I have to have my favorite fast-food meal—a burger, fries, and a chocolate shake—right now, to the point that I'll drive out of my way to get it.*

   ☐ *I'm upset when I feel the need to hide my "guilty pleasure" foods or lie to family and friends.*

   ☐ *What upsets me most is when I eat way too much dessert—a whole bag of cookies or a whole carton of ice cream—in one sitting, without stopping.*

   ☐ Other _____

   _____

2. Now think back to your most recent episode of this behavior and describe what happened. (Example: *I got home from dropping my kids off at school and next thing I knew, I was in the kitchen eating a large bag of chips. Before I realized it, the bag was almost empty.*)

_____

_____

_____

3. Think back to earlier in the day, before you did this behavior (or you may need to go back even further) and see if you can identify anything that might have triggered this episode. (Example: *When I dropped my kids off at school, my son's teacher pulled me aside to tell me about problems he was having at school, and asked if "everything was okay at home."*)

_____

_____

_____

4. Remember what you were feeling before you had the behavior and write down all the emotions you can remember, as well as any thoughts, fears, or judgments associated with those emotions. (Example: *I remember feeling frustrated and guilty. I know that my food addiction keeps me from being more aware of what's happening in my son's life.*)

_____

_____

_____

_____

_____

_____

5. Next, think of another episode of the same behavior you described in question 1. What triggered *that* episode? See if you can identify any similarities between these two situations. I've listed some questions below to get you started:

Did both situations make you feel the same emotions? (Example: *I felt guilty in both.*)

_____

_____

_____

Did you have similar body sensations? (Example: *I felt butterflies in my stomach and my face felt hot in both.*)

_____

_____

_____

Did you have similar thoughts about each situation? (Example: *I felt like I had let someone down, or that I was a failure, in both.*)

_____

_____

_____

Below, list any other insights you may have about the early warning signs of your food addiction behaviors:

_____

_____

_____

_____

If you can identify these early warning signs—the emotions, body sensations, and thoughts that happen before your food addiction behavior, you have a better chance of stopping or preventing the behavior in the future.

STEP 2: FINDING YOUR VALUES

The key to making a different choice is to be able to accept the moment. In order to accept the moment, you actually have to get to know yourself through your feelings. Rather than trying to push down your emotions with food, you can perhaps envision inviting those feelings to sit across from you.

In chapter 5, you learned about body sensations and about how the emotional soup can drive your behaviors. Now you can practice using your body sensations to identify your emotions and connect them with your behaviors. Instead of trying to avoid situations that you know will bring up emotions, you can learn how to experience your emotions without having to act on them—or at least not act on them right away. If you are like most individuals with food addiction, you may not be aware that emotions are like clues to what your values are, what your truth is. If you follow the breadcrumbs of your emotions, you can find out what the truth is. Behind every strong emotion is something you feel strongly enough about to get emotional. Let's look at Christie's story to understand this more.

Christie came to my office one day and immediately upon sitting down began to express how upset and angry she was. When I asked her to tell me why, she described a confrontation she'd had with her mother in which, she said, her mother was trying to give her parenting advice. Her mother was concerned that Christie's son was starting to gain weight. But before her mother could get very far with her advice, Christie burst into tears and left.

What was going on in this situation? On a superficial level, Christie obviously connected her own food and eating problems with the comment her mother made about her son's weight. But when she looked a little deeper and asked herself what overarching value she felt she was not in alignment with, she gained much more insight. Christie was able to realize that one of her values was being a good mother. When her mother made the observation that her son was gaining weight, unconsciously Christie interpreted her comment as meaning *I'm not a good mother.* Another way of phrasing this would be *I'm not in alignment with my value of being a good mother.* This feeling could also be triggered by a teacher saying her son wasn't doing well in school, or by many other situations. Often, when you experience strong emotions, there is an underlying value that is not in alignment with your actions.

Going from a strong emotion directly to bingeing or obsessing about food is often an automatic response. The key to changing this is uncoupling the emotion from the behavior—opening up enough space for you to identify the value you want to refocus on. To do that requires that you stay mindful every step of the way. There are skills you can use to do this.

EXERCISE:
Uncoupling Skills

1. Review the exercise in step 1 and see if you can make a list of values that are most important to you. I've listed some to get you started:

    ☐ *I value spending time with my family. So when I'm not being present with them (obsessing about food or my body), I feel guilty or ashamed.*

    ☐ *I value being kind to others. So when I'm irritable or mean-spirited (when I've had a binge, my self-esteem is low, and I'm beating myself up), I feel sad or afraid that my food addiction is out of control.*

    ☐ *I value being conscientious at work. So when I'm slacking off because I have low energy from not eating all day, or when I've binged in secret on foods brought in for everyone, I feel shame, guilt, and embarrassment.*

    ☐ *I value* _____.

    So when I (act against my values by) _____

    _____ , *I feel* (strong negative emotions)

    _____.

2. Identify techniques you can use to create some distance from these strong emotions so you can work on realigning with your values:

    ☐ *I will write an affirmation that states my value and use it when I feel the emotions in my example above. (Example: I am not a perfect mother, but every day I am actively working on being the best mother I can be.) My affirmation is:*

    _____

    _____

    _____

    ☐ *Every night before bedtime, I will write in my journal at least one thing I have done that supports my values. (Example: I was completely present while reading a bedtime story to my son.)*

☐ *I will make a vision board that illustrates what it would look like to live from one of my most important values.* (A vision board is a sign on which you can display a way you want to be in your life. You can use poster board or a corkboard, and attach magazine clippings, drawings, sayings, or whatever helps you illustrate the particular value. For example, a vision board about being a good parent might show a picture of you walking with your son, going to his baseball game, or volunteering at his school. It may show a picture of a peaceful family meal. Use it as a way to project and illustrate what your values mean to you. You can keep a picture of your vision board on your smart phone to look at when strong emotions threaten to overtake you. Or use the image as the screen saver on your computer.)

☐ Other techniques for creating space between your strong emotions and behaviors:

_____

_____

_____

_____

_____

_____

STEP 3: PRACTICING ACCEPTANCE

When you practice acceptance, you need to identify the value that your behavior is contradicting and then stop judging yourself for your behavior not being in alignment with this value. Acceptance is not about saying something is right or wrong, or that an event should or shouldn't have happened. Worrying about the future or dwelling on the past is what causes most of our suffering. You may spend a lot of time rehashing the past, evaluating your behavior or the behavior of someone else. Unfortunately, this doesn't change what has already happened. Accepting your situation doesn't change what has happened either. But it gives you space to heal. It doesn't prevent you from protecting yourself in the future or evaluating situations you are faced with now. Both of these skills can coexist with acceptance.

Think of acceptance as a choice between two paths: you can go down the path that makes you feel worse and leads to a binge or to more obsessive thoughts, or in the moment you can choose another path—one that lessens suffering. When you make this choice, you are choosing to accept only *this* present moment. This is similar to one of the principles from the 12-Step traditions—that you practice sobriety "one day at a time." The next exercise will give you a chance to practice acceptance.

EXERCISE:
Closing the Door on Suffering

Find a comfortable place to sit. Place your feet flat on the floor. Uncross your arms, hands, and legs. Take three deep breaths—breathing in through your nose and out through your mouth. Imagine that, with each breath, your body is becoming very heavy and relaxed, as if it is melting into the chair.

When you feel relaxed and calm, imagine one of the triggering situations you listed in the exercise above. Notice the thoughts and emotions and body sensations you experienced. Take a deep breath and ask yourself what value is beneath these emotions. Affirm this value. You may say something like, "I value being a good mother," for example. Sit with that feeling that this value is important to you. Breathe in the joy that living in your value brings to you. Imagine yourself doing activities that support your value. Now take another deep breath and say to yourself, "All is well" or, "Everything is perfect in this moment." You may feel another emotion or thought begin to argue with you. Again, take a deep breath and say, "All is well."

Repeat this at least a few times; then allow all your thoughts to drift away from you. You can imagine writing your thoughts or emotions in the sand on a beach and watching the tide come in and wash them away. As you see this, remind yourself, "All is well in this moment." Continue to focus on your breathing and allow your body to stay relaxed. You can also imagine seeing the value you identified being written in stone on a large rock on the beach. Sit by this rock as you watch the waves come in, washing away the pain and suffering.

When you are ready, return to an awareness of the room you are in. Look around you and again repeat to yourself, "All is well." Take another deep breath, smile, open up your heart, and go back to your day.

Cultivating mindfulness is one way to detoxify your mind. Practicing the skill of acceptance allows you to reduce some of the emotional toxicity that may be fueling your food addiction.

Wrap-up

You have now learned about the emotional, biological, and environmental causes that may contribute to your food addiction. Even if you can't find a reason for your obsessive focus on food and your body size, you may be very aware of the suffering your food addiction has caused. The steps you've learned about in this chapter require a willingness on your part to let go of that suffering. They require the willingness to connect with your body in a different way and listen to its wisdom about what it wants to eat. Most of all, they require a willingness to be more aware of your emotions, thoughts, and body sensations, and how your body reacts to the food you give it.

These steps may seem monumental—perhaps too overwhelming or frightening to even contemplate. If you give up or let go of your food addiction, how will you comfort yourself when you're upset? How will you have a break from life without using food? Don't try to figure it all out now. Just ask yourself if you are willing to move in that direction. If you are, the next chapters will help support you in your recovery from food addiction. Each chapter in part 3 offers tools to help you continue your journey in finding freedom from food addiction.

PART 3

Thriving in Recovery

In part 2, you learned about the Five Levels of Healing from food addiction. You can use these levels as a road map in your recovery. Starting with changing superficial behaviors, you can move through the different levels—the emotional soup, body sensations, core beliefs, and soul satisfaction. It is important that you focus first on changing your behaviors so that you are not distracted by your obsessive thoughts about food and your body. As you move through the levels, you will notice that your emotions, your body sensations, and even your beliefs will begin to shift. As these levels change, your experience of soul satisfaction will grow and you will find yourself being more committed to doing things that strengthen your recovery, rather than things that weaken your recovery.

In part 2, you also learned about physical problems in the body that could create or worsen food cravings and obsessive thoughts about food. Paying attention to how your gut works and how your body responds to what you eat will give you valuable information aimed at improving your health. In the last chapter of part 2, you learned how to break the hold that food has on your life and how to free yourself from the prison of your thoughts and cravings through mindful awareness.

Part 3 is all about thriving in recovery. For many people, especially those with addictions, recovery simply means abstaining from their drug of choice to break its hold. In process addictions like food or eating addictions, you cannot abstain from food. But you can learn to abstain from your behaviors, as discussed in the Five Levels in chapter 5. This is an important first step, but only a first step. Recovery is more than just no longer eating impulsively or obsessing about food. A deeper definition of recovery should involve having an improved quality of life. This may include having the energy to do the things you want to do, being less stressed in your life, having a kinder relationship with your body, and building a community of people who are supportive of your recovery.

In part 3, you will learn how to expand your experience of recovery and skills that will enable you to live from a more peaceful, less chaotic and obsessed place. This includes reducing the "noise" in your life that is caused by stress and toxic emotions. In later chapters, you will be able to learn ways to address your body image concerns, and you will learn skills you can use to continue your journey toward nourishing your body, mind, and spirit without restriction, addiction, or fear. The last chapter in part 3 will help you to build a stronger foundation for your recovery by learning about how social support can help you heal from reward deficiency syndrome and food addiction. The focus of part 3 is to help you move toward actually making the changes you need to make. Let's get started!

CHAPTER 7

Stress Management

Jeremy worked for a high-end marketing firm and his job was a big source of stress in his life. Long hours at work and frequent client dinners left him exhausted and made it difficult for him to control his eating. Stress made his obsessive thoughts about food and fear of gaining more weight worse. When he came home, he was lonely and tired but couldn't get to sleep. When he couldn't sleep, he would go back downstairs and snack in front of the television. He gravitated toward eating large bags of chips with salsa (justifying to himself that "at least I'm eating some vegetables.") He didn't have time or energy to go to the gym, and anyway, he was embarrassed to even try to get into his workout clothes.

He found himself gaining even more weight when his partner of five years left him after admitting to having an affair with a coworker. Jeremy also began drinking more heavily after this happened. He had difficulty sleeping and his weight continued to increase until he found himself having to buy new suits in a larger size than ever before. He wasn't sure if he was depressed, but he felt down most days and didn't look forward to anything in his life.

Jeremy knew he was at his lowest point in life when he crossed the street to avoid running into an old friend he hadn't seen since he'd gotten so fat. Later that night, his friend called him and asked him if he was "okay." Jeremy broke down in tears of shame and guilt and also of appreciation that someone cared enough about him to ask. His friend referred him to the Anchor Program, and Jeremy made an appointment for the following week.

In the program, Jeremy worked on being able to manage his emotions without always using food. He began to use an online app to keep track of his eating and to monitor his stress level. He also used a different app that taught him small, easy ways he could be more present, and he even began to meditate for five to ten minutes a day. He also worked on the grief from breaking up with his partner. He started keeping a journal and spending more time with friends. He took supplements to help him sleep and to help his body deal with stress better. He learned how to take more time for himself and got back into taking walks with his dog. He began to feel less overwhelmed and he found his mood gradually improving.

In chapter 6, you learned how to break the hold food has on your life. Part of why food may have such power in your life is that you may be using food to deal with emotional ups and downs and with stress. You may recognize that your food choices change when you're upset or stressed out, just as they did for Jeremy when he experienced work stress, and after his breakup. You may also find yourself eating more or being more focused on food when under stress. In this chapter, you will learn more about why stress management is so important for those with food addiction and about tools you can use to manage your stress and emotions in a way that is less food-obsessed.

Stress, Eating, and Food Addiction

Stress has tremendous influence on your health and well-being. If you have a food addiction or other eating addiction, you know that you spend lots of your mental time and energy obsessing about food and your body. The problem with a stress-filled life is that it may affect your food choices and eating patterns, and that stress can be one of the reasons why your emotions are on a roller coaster—another factor that can lead to overeating, bingeing, or using food to distract or numb yourself. Here are a few facts about stress and eating behaviors to ponder:

- Under stress, emotional eaters consume more sweet, high-fat foods and more high-calorie meals than normal eaters (Oliver et al. 2000; Dallman 2010). While about 30 percent of people under stress will lose their appetite and actually lose weight, the majority of people tend to overeat and gain weight when under stress (Adam and Epel 2007).

- Stress and its effect on the brain reward system, along with repeated consumption of highly palatable foods, may promote compulsive overeating.

- Stress is a critical factor in the development of addictive behaviors, and may also contribute to relapse from addictions (Sinha 2008).

- The increase in obesity in the United States may have been exacerbated by the prevalence of chronic stress and repeated attempts at dieting (Adam and Epel 2007).

- Stress, depression, and anxiety are highly associated with—and may trigger—addiction-like eating behavior.

- People who are trying to control their weight (via dieting, appetite suppressants, or excessive exercise) consistently overeat or binge when under stress, leading to weight gain (Greeno and Wing 1994; Chua et al. 2004).

- Weight regain six months following successful weight loss is strongly associated with eating in response to stress or negative mood (Elfhag and Rossner 2005).

As you can see, stress can intensify your struggles with food and your body, and obsessing about food or your body can in turn be its own source of stress. It's a vicious cycle that can leave you feeling discouraged. Learning to manage stress is the key to breaking the cycle.

Sources of Stress

Stress is your response to highly challenging or overwhelming life events. Essentially, the body's "fight, flight, or freeze" reaction is triggered. This may occur even though the circumstances are not literally life-threatening. Your mind interprets the events as dangerous in some way, and then your body responds as if that were truly the case. The stress-provoking situation may affect the body, the mind, or the spirit. Common sources of stress can be categorized as follows (American Institute of Stress, N.D.):

1. Emotional experiences. Events such as interpersonal conflict, loss of a relationship, loss of a job, or death of a loved one can all trigger strong negative emotions that cause stress. Sometimes unpleasant emotions such as sadness or anxiety arise without a clear triggering event. Your own internal reactions to these emotions can be a further source of stress. For instance, if you feel angry over a job loss for an extended period of time, you may then judge yourself for feeling angry, wondering, *Why can't I just let it go?* That self-judgment can become an additional source of stress.

2. Physiological stressors (relating to the body's functions). Simply facing challenging physical conditions can be stressful. Conditions such as hunger, food deprivation or overeating and bingeing, inadequate sleep, hormonal changes of puberty or menopause, and aging are all potential sources of stress. Additionally, you may find it stressful to experience frequent colds or flu or to learn that you have a more severe illness (Yau and Potenza 2013).

3. Environmental stressors. It's stressful to be exposed to pollution, noise, traffic, extreme weather changes, and toxins in the air and in products you use.

4. Mental activity. Your mind provides a constant stream of thoughts interpreting the events you experience. As you assess the meanings of situations and the motivations of people in your environment, the nature of your interpretations greatly affects the level of stress you experience. You can choose to judge what is

happening, label the situation as negative, or make dire predictions about the future—any of which can lead to greater stress. Or you may respond to events with a calm, accepting attitude, in which case you'll experience life in a more positive or optimistic light and lessen your stress.

It's important to note that mental and emotional stresses arise largely because the demands of the situation exceed your perceived ability to cope. In other words, you believe you are trapped or won't be able to resolve the situation successfully. It's inherently stressful to be in such a bind. While there's not much you can do about physiological and environmental stressors like illness or pollution, you do have a fair amount of influence over your mental and emotional reactions to events. By learning to treat yourself with kindness and keep an open mind, you can significantly reduce your own experience of stress.

How Stress Affects the Body and Mind

During stressful times, the body is always trying to achieve stability. Changes in your mood, sleep patterns, and eating habits are all attempts at reaching a more stable state. Very severe stress or chronic stress that lasts a long time can cause wear and tear on the body, making it more difficult to reach stability, and causing infections, diseases, depression, and addictive behaviors (McEwen 2007). High levels of stress are strongly associated with weight gain, especially among people who are already overweight or who binge eat (Block et al. 2009). If you gain weight under stress, it may be because stress changes your metabolism (how your body processes the foods you are eating), makes you more likely to choose foods that are higher in sugar, salt, or fat, or makes you snack more (Dallman et al. 2005; Oliver et al. 2000). If you are under stress, you may also skip meals, restrict what you eat, or consume more fast food (Torres and Nowson 2007; Gluck et al. 2004). Besides changes in your eating patterns under stress, you may also lose sleep, exercise less, and drink more alcoholic beverages—all of which may cause a worsening of your food addiction behaviors and weight gain. If you are a woman, you may be more likely to turn to food during stressful times, whereas men may be more likely to smoke or drink alcohol. In African-Americans, feeling stressed out is associated with more emotional eating (eating foods high in sugar and fat), haphazard meal planning (leading to eating more high-fat foods), and snacking on sweets (Sims et al. 2008).

Your body responds to stress by initially producing adrenaline and then, if the stress continues, producing cortisol. Having higher cortisol levels in response to stress may make you more likely to snack in response to daily stress compared with people who produce less cortisol. Cortisol also increases the tendency to overeat. This does not mean that relieving stress by eating comfort foods once in a while will make you fat. However, if food is your main way of coping with stress, this pattern can lead to obesity and exacerbate food addiction behaviors.

There is overlap between the stress pathways in the brain that motivate you to eat certain foods under stress and the part of the brain that deals with emotions (called the limbic system). What this means is that stress and negative emotions decrease emotional and behavioral control and increase impulsivity, making it more likely that you will binge on your drug of choice—alcohol for the alcoholic, or food for the person with food addiction (Hays and Roberts 2008; Sinha et al. 2009).

Another effect of stress that is worse in those with food addiction, drug addiction, or alcohol addiction is the effect of stress on the brain reward system. Stress causes a decrease in dopamine in the brain. Initially, when you eat comfort foods or other highly palatable foods, you may feel a sense of calming or a sense of pleasure caused by a spike in dopamine in the brain. However, repeated consumption of these foods has the opposite effect and dopamine release is reduced. As dopamine release is reduced, you will experience more cravings and may actually be compelled to repeatedly eat the foods you are craving to keep from feeling bad (Parylak et al. 2011; Volkow and O'Brien 2007). This process is similar to what happens with drugs of abuse that initially people take for the "high" but over time they have to keep taking to avoid the pain of low moods, anxiety, and other withdrawal symptoms.

You may still be unconvinced that stress has anything to do with your food addiction. However, besides the research listed earlier in this chapter, stress reduction has been shown in studies to be one of the contributing factors to being able to maintain weight loss over a long period of time (Wing and Phelan 2005; Franz et al. 2007). Knowing how stress affects you physically, mentally, and emotionally will enable you to begin to change how you deal with it. There are many ways to improve how you cope with stress. Just as each of us perceives and reacts to stress in different ways, there is no single stress-reduction strategy that works for everyone. Below, I'll discuss some ways you can reduce your level of stress, or cope more effectively with it.

Building Resilience to Stress

Since you can't really avoid stress in your life, nor would you want to (remember, there are many positive life experiences that can be stressful, too), it's important to become more resilient to stress. Resilience describes the ability to bounce back from stress and to thrive and survive despite the stress in your life. Being resilient doesn't mean you don't feel stress or difficulty in your life. And resilience is not something you're born with. It involves changing your thoughts, managing your emotions, and learning new ways to cope with stress.

Staying in Good Physical Condition

It may seem obvious, but it is worth mentioning that being physically healthy helps you combat stress. Being well nourished, getting enough sleep, having a strong support system, and exercising regularly can all help you improve or maintain good physical health. During periods of high or chronic stress it is also a good idea to limit your intake of alcohol and nicotine. Nutrition and social support will be covered in later chapters. Sleep and exercise are so important in combating stress that they deserve some further discussion here.

SLEEP

Sleep is a necessary function in your life—even though, for most people, sleep is the thing they do *after* they've attended to everything that is "important." Adults who sleep fewer than eight hours a night report higher stress levels, less motivation, more irritability, lower energy levels, and less exercise than those who sleep at least eight hours a night. Chronic sleep deprivation contributes to obesity, high blood pressure, diabetes, and addictions. Poor sleep may result in an increase in food cravings, and not sleeping well may leave you too tired to burn off extra calories that are consumed. Sleep helps balance appetite by controlling the hormones ghrelin and leptin, which regulate your feelings of hunger and fullness. (American Psychological Association 2014).

To improve your sleep, the best place to start is with the general guidelines for good sleep hygiene:

- Go to bed at the same time and get up at the same time whenever possible

- Establish a regular wind-down routine (such as taking a warm bath, reading a relaxing book, or listening to soothing music)

- Avoid stimulants such as alcohol, caffeine, and tobacco close to bedtime

- Use your bed only for sleeping and sex (in other words, don't work or watch TV in bed)

- Keep your bedroom dark and not too hot or too cold

- Use a white-noise machine or app if you live in a noisy neighborhood

Following these guidelines is worth the effort. Getting a good night's sleep is extremely important to your overall health and well-being, and to your recovery from food addiction.

EXERCISE

You may be used to thinking of exercise only in the context of trying to lose weight, and exercise may or may not be your favorite thing to do. If you are lucky enough to have a positive view of physical activity, that's great! Keep going! If not, first I'd like to let you know that this book is not about making you want to exercise for weight reduction. What's important in the context of food addiction recovery is that regular physical activity may protect you against the negative emotional effects of stress (Childs and de Wit 2014). To stay physically strong and build stress resilience, any kind of physical activity is useful. Don't get stuck limiting yourself to exercises that you've been told will help with weight. Instead, think of things you like to do, ways you like to move your body. This could be with walking, dancing, jumping rope, swimming, biking, or many, many other activities. Try to recall the ways you enjoyed being active as a child and start there. Remember to tailor your exercise to how your body is feeling under stress. If you're feeling jittery or irritable, you may feel like engaging in an aggressively active sport, such as running or tennis. If your body is exhausted, you might consider a restorative yoga class, swimming, or a walk. No matter what you choose, remind yourself that you are doing this for your health, and to help you cope better with stress.

Managing Emotions

It's a given that stressful events in life can bring up lots of emotions—sometimes both positive and negative ones at the same time. People who are resilient to stress tend to be more optimistic and have more positive than negative emotions overall. You may have noticed that negative emotions tend to make you want to attack or escape. Positive emotions, on the other hand, tend to help broaden your outlook and allow you to be more creative and open to problem solving. If you are a person with reward deficiency syndrome (RDS), you may find yourself reacting more negatively in stressful situations than other people do. What can you do about this? It's very important to be aware of when you're experiencing negative emotions, rather than thinking, *That's just how I am.* Here are some techniques to help shift your emotional state:

1. Apply humor. Research has shown that humor can improve depressive symptoms by fostering a more positive outlook and by attracting social support (Kuiper and McHale 2009). Interestingly, for those with RDS, humor has been shown to activate essential parts of the brain that make up the dopamine reward system (Blum et al. 2015). When you're feeling down, try watching a funny movie or show, reading a humorous book, or spending time with a friend who has a good sense of humor.

2. Take a break. Finding a way to unhook from your emotions may be helpful in coping with stressful situations. You can do this by using one of these techniques:

   a. Belly breathing: Inhale slowly and deeply. Push your belly out as you breathe in. Hold your breath for five seconds. Then exhale slowly, thinking *calm*, or *peace*. Repeat five times. You can also imagine "breathing in peace" and "breathing out stress" or "breathing out fear."

   b. Guided imagery for relaxation. (A guided imagery exercise is available at http://www.newharbinger.com/32097.)

Supplements to Support Your Body in Managing Stress

If you'd like to explore the use of supplements, please get clearance from your health care practitioner and don't start several new supplements at the same time. Start with one and then add a second. That way, if you have any negative reactions you will be able to identify which supplement was the source of the side effect (http://data.integrativepro.com/downloads/hpa-nutritional-therapies-guide.pdf).

To help relieve anxiety and feeling stressed out (tired but wired):

- Ashwagandha—may lower cortisol and help with mood; modulates hormonal changes due to stress. Take 200–400 mg daily.

- L-theanine—promotes muscle relaxation and reduces anxiety. This is the amino acid in green tea. Take 50–200 mg daily in divided doses.

- Phosphatidylserine—supports cognitive ability (memory, judgment), enhances exercise capacity, and reduces stress. Take 50–100 mg at bedtime.

- Lavender oil—can be used in an aerosolizer, or by applying a few drops to your pillowcase at night, to reduce anxiety.

For low mood, low energy, and problems with memory and concentration:

- *Rhodiola rosea*—reduces fatigue and improves mood. Start with 50 mg twice daily and increase to 200–400 mg a day.

- Siberian ginseng—increases resistance to stress and helps to regulate the neurotransmitters that control mood. Take 150–300 mg daily in pill form, or drink ginseng tea.

For chronic or long-term stress:

The following supplements work well if you've had chronic or very severe stress and find yourself not being able to cope. These work for exhaustion, especially at the end of your day; emotional hypersensitivity; trouble falling asleep; and trouble staying asleep.

- B vitamins—necessary for the production of many of the neurotransmitters (such as serotonin and dopamine) that affect mood. A B-complex vitamin may help restore sleep and improve your body's response to stress. Take a B-complex with methylated folate and B_{12} every morning.

- Deglycyrrhizinated licorice—helps your body with digestion, boosts the immune system, and helps with body aches and pains. Take 150–300 mg daily.

- Melatonin—promotes better sleep quality and helps you fall asleep faster. Take 3 mg at bedtime.

- 5-hydroxytryptophan (5-HTP)—a serotonin precursor that may help restore dreams and deepen sleep, and may improve mood. Take 50–100 mg at bedtime.

Caution: If you are taking prescription medications (including antidepressants), if you are pregnant or nursing, or if you have any medical problems, please consult your health care provider before taking any supplements.

Changing Your Thoughts

You may not realize that you have the ability to change your thoughts, or you may not have made the connection between your thoughts and how they affect your mood and eating behaviors. For a moment, consider seeing your supervisor from work walking down the street with a very negative expression on her face. She barely speaks to you as you pass by. Your first thought may be, *I wonder what I've done wrong? What if it's something at work and she tells my boss? How will I keep my job if this happens?* This may then lead to feeling bad about yourself and wracking your brain to figure out what you did. Or you may have the thought: *Who does she think she is, snubbing me? I can't do anything right! Every time I get comfortable in a job, someone turns against me!* Again, this thought can lead to a whole host of other thoughts—all of them negative. Imagine how all these negative thoughts make you feel. You may feel sad, angry, or afraid. Now, fast-forward to the next day, when you see your supervisor in the grocery store. She comes up to you and says, "I'm so sorry about yesterday. When I saw you, I had just found out that my mother was diagnosed with breast cancer. I was a mess." This is an example of how your beliefs about a situation can sometimes feel more real than the actual truth.

Think about all the times in your life when this has happened: an argument with a sibling, a tense meeting at work, fearful thoughts about your children. All of the thoughts associated with these situations often take on a life of their own, triggering emotions and then behaviors that can exacerbate your stress and your food addiction. Things happen in your life that you react to, and these reactions can lead you back to your food addiction as a way to cope.

Your thoughts have a huge impact on how you deal with stress, and when you're not coping well it may be because of the following assumptions, or "trigger thoughts" (McKay and Rogers 2000).

1. You believe you've been harmed or victimized.

2. You believe that something was done deliberately to harm you.

3. You believe that you are right about the situation and any other interpretation is wrong.

Whenever you are in a situation and you have a thought that you're being victimized or that someone's out to get you, this thought can trigger a whole cascade of other thoughts, judgments, and behaviors that end up making you feel worse instead of better. One way to manage your thoughts is to reevaluate and find positive meaning in a situation that has been stressful for you. Resilient people tend to be able to view harmful and stressful events in a less threatening light, and doing this tends to result in a more positive outcome (Southwick et al. 2005). This kind of reevaluation involves:

1. Finding a greater appreciation for your personal strengths

2. Realizing that your life experiences are making you wiser

3. Recognizing that life is very precious

4. Reordering your priorities

5. Opening up to acceptance

This final strategy—cultivating acceptance, which was discussed in the previous chapter—is extremely powerful, yet it's not always easy to do. Acceptance is especially important when you are faced with a situation that you cannot change. If you think about it, events and circumstances are stressful only when you resist them or try to avoid them—in other words, when you have a judgment about what is happening (it's good or bad, right or wrong) and you believe that it should be some other way, not that way.

You may think of this way of thinking as the most natural thing in the world. Of course it's awful to be stuck in a traffic jam or to be subjected to the constant barking of a neighbor's dog. Of course it's painful to be criticized by your partner or be disappointed that your body doesn't look like you think it should. Buddhist philosophy states that while pain is part of the human condition (the Christian version is: "everyone has their cross to bear"), suffering is not. Suffering is caused by nonacceptance of pain, or by wanting things to be different than they are—a desire that is sometimes called craving. When you don't accept yourself or other people or your surroundings the way they are, there is suffering, and the stress attached to the situation worsens. If you choose to surrender to the reality of the situation, there may be pain, but there will not be as much suffering. Here's an example: The death of a loved one is a very traumatic event for many people, but not one that can be changed. Holding onto a belief that somehow your anger can change the situation only causes more suffering and stress. Acceptance is not the same as being resigned or giving up. It simply means that you accept the reality of the situation as it is; you accept the facts. You may have your own opinions about the facts, and you certainly may have emotions about the facts, but neither changes the facts. When you're faced with conditions or events that are not fully within your control, acceptance can be the most useful tool in your stress reduction tool kit.

Becoming more resilient to stress involves attending to your physical health—possibly with the use of supplements—as well as managing your thoughts and emotions. In the next exercise, you will have the chance to incorporate some of the coping strategies presented in this chapter into your own personal coping plan that you can put into action. (A downloadable version of this exercise is available at http://www.newharbinger.com/32097.)

EXERCISE:
Your Personal Stress Coping Plan

Use this exercise to develop your personal stress coping plan. In each of the following categories, check off one or more actions you plan to take to improve how you manage stress, and fill in the blanks with more specifics where appropriate. Remember not to be overly ambitious. Take small, practical steps that you can actually do. You can come back to this plan over time and add or take out things that you want to try, or that have worked or not worked. Think of it as a road map to better life stress management.

When under stress I will take care of my physical health by:

Monitoring or reducing my intake of alcohol. (Example: *I will pay attention to when I'm drinking for emotional reasons, won't drink alone, and will set a drink limit.*)

_____

_____

Monitoring or reducing my use of nicotine. (Example: *I won't increase the amount I'm smoking when I feel stressed.*)

_____

_____

Improving my sleep hygiene by changing the following: (See list of sleep hygiene recommendations above.)

_____

_____

Moving my body by: (Examples: *doing some stretching, going to a yoga class, taking a walk, going to Pilates class, kayaking*)

_____

_____

Taking a rest by: (Examples: *sitting outside in nature, walking on the beach, listening to music*)

_____

_____

When under stress I will practice managing my emotions by:

Using humor.

_____

_____

Practicing breathing techniques.

_____

_____

Taking a meditation class or listening to a guided imagery recording.

_____

_____

Other:

_____

_____

When I am under stress, I will consider the following supplements, after getting clearance from my health care provider. (Copy from the list of supplements earlier in this chapter the ones you'd like to try. Remember to start only one supplement at a time.)

1. _____

2. _____

3. _____

4. _____

5. _____

When I am under stress and I find my thoughts taking over my mind, I will.

1. Try to find a greater appreciation for my personal strengths. (Example: *I will stop discounting what a strong woman I am and will remind myself that I am kind and generous—values that are important to me.*)

_____

_____

_____

2. Work on realizing that my life experiences are making me wiser. Here are some of the ways in which I have become wiser: (Example: *After the breakup with his boyfriend, Jeremy was able to realize that his relationship was not a healthy one. As he became more committed to himself and his recovery, he was able to use this experience to help him pick someone he could be in a healthier relationship with.*)

_____

_____

_____

3. Encourage myself to recognize that life is very precious. (Example: *When I think of how much time and energy I put into thinking about what I shouldn't be eating, I will remind myself I am human and I deserve to eat good, enjoyable food and that I'm still learning what that means for me.*)

_____

_____

_____

4. Make a list of the pros and cons of what I consider important in my life, reordering my priorities if needed. (Example: *I always put myself last and take care of other people before I do what I need or want to do. This causes more stress in my life.*)

List a behavior you want to consider for reprioritization. Then list the pros and cons of making it a higher priority.

Behavior: _____

_____

Pros: _____

_____

Cons: _____

_____

Behavior: _____

_____

Pros: _____

_____

Cons: _____

_____

5. Open up to acceptance.

Where in your life are you resisting accepting things the way they are?

(Example: *Jeremy had a hard time accepting that his partner had broken up with him. He kept thinking that he could change the situation and they would get back together.*)

_____

_____

_____

What are your values about this situation? (Example: *Jeremy realized he wanted a partner who was supportive and not as negative as his previous partner.*)

_____

_____

_____

What would it take for you to accept the situation? (Example: *Jeremy realized that his fear of being alone was what kept him going back into unhealthy relationships. He was able to work in therapy on this fear so that he could feel comfortable with his decision.*)

_____

_____

_____

_____

As you learned more about the various ways to manage stress—by responding differently to thoughts, managing strong emotions, and taking good care of yourself physically—did you notice one particular area that stood out? Perhaps you realized that self-critical thoughts, plus your judgment of yourself for having those thoughts, are your own greatest source of stress. If this is the case, you may find it helpful to work on being more present in the here and now and extending more kindness to yourself. Maybe your main source of stress is your mind's tendency to assume that minor frustrations are going to have terrible consequences, in which case it can be liberating to remind yourself: *Don't sweat the small stuff.* If you feel stressed mainly in your relationships with other people, you may find it freeing to work on letting old grudges go and not taking things so personally. Or maybe you've come to see that your experiences of stress are worsened mainly by poor physical self-care, in which case the key might be to cultivate new habits of well-being, such as taking a walk at lunchtime, creating a soothing bedtime routine, or taking supplements that help your body bounce back from life's challenges. Take the time to build your resilience to stress in the way that works best for you. And when the going gets tough—as it occasionally will—keep your eye on the things that really matter to you.

Wrap-up

Stress can motivate you to do great things, or it can wear you down and leave you exhausted. If you have an eating or food addiction, you may have already noticed the effect that stress has when you use food as your primary coping mechanism. In this chapter, you've learned how stress can cause wear and tear on your body and how it can exacerbate your obsessive thoughts and behaviors around food. You've also learned ways to cope better with stress. By using your personal stress coping plan as a road map, you can gradually put in place and practice new skills that will give you a better handle on the stress that life brings.

In chapter 8, you will learn about how to address any body image issues that may keep you stuck in the vicious circle of trying to fix your body in order to feel better in your life.

CHAPTER 8

Putting an End to Body Hatred

Ariel reported that she remembered being unhappy with her body from about age eleven, when she started to go through puberty much earlier than the other kids in her class. By age twelve, she was already five foot eight, and she felt huge compared with her friends. She had breasts before anyone else and was teased by the boys in her class at recess. She just felt "huge" and "gross." She remembers sitting between her two friends in gym class and looking down at her legs, comparing them with the girls' on either side of her and saying to herself, "My thighs are huge!" Even though her friends eventually went through the same changes, she never got over this feeling of being bigger than everyone else, and the sense of not belonging.

To compensate for feeling so big, even though her weight was normal for her height, Ariel began to avoid eating foods that she thought were bad for her and cycling through one diet after another in high school to try to lose weight. She would lose weight and then regain the weight, and she could never find a weight at which she was less dissatisfied with her body. She also started bingeing on the foods that she was depriving herself of. In college, she started drinking more heavily, and she noticed that when she would drink she felt like she could also eat whatever she wanted—which led to binges on junk foods and sweets. When her roommates asked her about foods that were missing from the kitchen (after she'd had a binge), she would make excuses about having to throw food out because it spoiled, for example. She was embarrassed by her binges but even more ashamed of her body. She tried exercising and restrictive diets, which were followed by more bingeing and self-recrimination.

This cycle continued into her early twenties, by which time Ariel really hated her body and felt that she was powerless in her attempts at finding a way to make her body look the way she wanted it to look. She was not overweight, but she felt that her dissatisfaction with her body made it difficult for her to be in intimate relationships, and her food obsessions led to low self-esteem. She couldn't seem to accept compliments from others, and she constantly berated herself for being so "huge."

In chapter 7, you learned how stress can be a trigger for food addiction, and you also learned ways to improve your ability to cope with stress. This chapter is all about your relationship with your body. Body image involves your perceptions, thoughts, and behaviors related to appearance. It can have an impact on your self-esteem and on your quality of life.

Body image is established usually by the age of six, at which age children are aware of how they look and of society's bias against certain body types. During adolescence, body image continues to change and develop. External factors such as trauma, cultural influences, media, relationships, and life experiences can also have an impact on body image (Birbeck and Drummond 2006; Bolton et al. 2010).

Individuals with food addiction (based on the Yale Food Addiction Scale, discussed in chapter 1) tend to have issues related to weight and body image. These include more significant anti-fat attitudes, feelings of shame about their bodies, and the internalization of negative stereotypes about weight (Burmeister et al. 2013). If you are overweight or obese, you may have experienced weight bias (or weight shaming) from employers, teachers, family members, health care providers, and others. Several studies document that often these anti-fat attitudes and weight shaming are seen as truth by individuals who themselves are obese or overweight—in other words, these views have been internalized.

If you have food addiction and also hate your body, you may feel that by engaging in negative self-talk about your body you are motivating yourself to lose weight. In other words, you may think that by calling yourself "fat" or "lazy," or "disgusting" you can force yourself to change your eating behaviors. Other commonly perceived stereotypes about fat people include that they have poor hygiene, are unintelligent, lack willpower, eat unhealthy foods, and are worthless. If you believe any of these stereotypes, you may be trying to whip yourself into shape by using negative feedback and negative self-talk. However, as one of my clients eventually realized, "You can't hate yourself thin." If this strategy were an effective one, the increase in weight-based stigmatization in our culture would have led to a decrease in obesity, rather than the significant increase seen over the past forty years. Research studies have shown that obese individuals who believe in weight-based stereotypes are in fact *less* likely to change their behaviors and more likely to binge eat (Puhl et al. 2007).

If self-hatred won't help you overcome your struggles with your eating and your weight, what will? The key is to understand the importance of your thoughts. When you understand what beliefs you hold about your body and how you formed those beliefs, you'll be in a position to form a new, mature, healthy view of your body. When you relate to your body in a new way, you will finally be free to live the life of your dreams.

Causes of Body Hatred

In order to change your feelings about your body, you'll need to understand how you formed those harsh, self-critical beliefs in the first place. Where does this body hatred come from? In this section, you'll learn more about the many causes of body dissatisfaction.

Social norms—and the extent to which you believe in them—are one major cause. Body dissatisfaction among girls tends to increase following puberty. Body dissatisfaction is also a concern among adolescent boys but tends to decrease during puberty. For both boys and girls, body hatred can lead to emotional distress and dramatic efforts to change appearance (such as steroid use or cosmetic surgery) along with eating disorders and depression. Often as girls mature, they become obsessed with being more attractive, and in western culture this means being thin. Boys, on the other hand, may be more focused on becoming bigger and more muscular, although there are some boys who also value being thin. How much a girl or boy buys into the need to be thin, or a boy buys into the need to be muscular, to be accepted will predict the level of body dissatisfaction, especially as a teenager.

Lack of social support can also be a risk factor for body hatred. Feeling that you are not fully accepted or loved by your family and friends makes it harder to love and accept yourself, especially when your body goes through changes. If, like Ariel, you matured early and were teased by peers or even by members of your own family, you are more likely to feel bad about your body than someone who received more support, especially if you are a girl. Social support, or lack of it, does not seem to have as great an effect on boys.

If you tend to be a perfectionist, this personality trait also puts you at higher risk for body hatred. Perfectionism, especially the fear of making mistakes and being judged by others, can lead you to attempt to create the perfect body, based on media images or other cultural ideals. As part of perfectionism, the need to be overly organized (be in control of your environment) may also promote body hatred, which might be explained by the need to control body appearance. And when one is not able to do this, it may lead to self-criticism and negative moods that are focused on the body (Wade and Tiggermann 2013).

One of the most common causes of body hatred stems from traumatic experiences. One in five women and one in seventy-one men will be raped in their lifetime (US Centers for Disease Control and Prevention 2012). Sexual assault at any time in your life can lead to feeling powerless or worthless. In an effort to cope, some people focus on controlling their bodies. Sexual trauma is more prevalent in the history of individuals with eating disorders than in those without. It is believed that when sexual trauma comes before an eating disorder, it contributes to the development of body dissatisfaction, shame, sexual problems, and fear of future sexual trauma. The eating disorder can be a way to cope with the trauma, or to regulate negative emotions (Madowitz et al. 2015). In African-American victims of trauma, body dissatisfaction and depression have been associated with the severity of both physical and sexual assault. In other words, the more severe the physical or sexual assault, the more likely the victim would experience body dissatisfaction and depression. The violation of trust that is often involved in sexual trauma also leads to body dissatisfaction (Weaver et al. 2014). Often victims of assault or abuse may not connect their past experiences with their current body hatred. That's because sexual trauma doesn't affect everyone the same way. It's very likely, however, that if you are experiencing body hatred and you've been a victim of sexual trauma, the trauma is a significant causative factor of your body image issues.

Other causes of body dissatisfaction include struggles with mood. Extreme measures to lose weight—such as recurrent dieting, binge eating, purging, fasting, or excessive exercise—are associated with emotional distress and feelings of guilt, frustration, or loss of control over one's eating. All of these feelings may foster body hatred. If you suffer from depression, you may have noticed an increase in body dissatisfaction, an increased focus on what you don't like about your body, and the tendency to make negative comparisons between your body and that of your peers or other family members. Boys with high levels of body dissatisfaction may also be more prone to depression, eating disorders, obesity, and drug abuse (Field et al. 2014).

You may be thinking, *If my thighs weren't so big, or (fill in the blank), I wouldn't hate my body.* But body hatred is not always associated with body weight, shape, or size, especially in boys. In one study, male adolescents who were most dissatisfied with their bodies were of no different weight than those who were happy with their bodies. This may mean that body dissatisfaction has more to do with how you perceive your weight than what you actually weigh (Bearman et al. 2006). If you hate your body, that feeling may be a cause of significant suffering in your life. You may struggle with making choices about what to wear, your thoughts about your body may make it difficult for you to enjoy being in social situations, and your body hatred may make it challenging for you to want to take care of your body. You may also want to blame your body for how it makes you feel.

Hopefully by reading this book, you've begun to change your perceptions about your body somewhat, and you may now be able to understand that it is your *perception* of your body that causes suffering. If your perception is that your body doesn't live up to whatever you would like your body to look like or what you feel is expected by society, then your perception is what needs to change, not your body. Your body is just the way it is and nothing will change by your berating, judging, and calling your body names. If you could "hate yourself thin" it would already have happened, don't you think? So let's focus on this perception of how your body doesn't live up to your expectations, and how that perception actually causes suffering in your life. In the next exercise, you will be able to explore some of the consequences of your body hatred.

EXERCISE:
How Your Body Hatred Affects Your Life

In this exercise, see if you can identify all the ways in which your hatred of your body limits or impacts your life as a whole.

1. When I go shopping for clothing, my hatred of my body causes:

   a. Feelings of _____

   _____

   b. Actions such as _____

   _____

   c. Limitations in my life such as _____

   _____

2. In my friendships my body hatred causes:

   a. Feelings of _____

   _____

   b. Actions such as _____

   _____

   c. Limitations in my life such as _____

   _____

3. In intimate relationships (or my desire for intimate relationships), my body hatred causes:

   a. Feelings of _____

   _____

   b. Actions such as _____

   _____

c. Limitations in my life such as _____
_____

4. When I am in social situations, my body hatred causes:

   a. Feelings of _____
_____

   b. Actions such as _____
_____

   c. Limitations in my life such as _____
_____

5. When I try to nurture my body, or think about nurturing my body (for example, with healthy eating), my body hatred causes:

   a. Feelings of _____
_____

   b. Actions such as _____
_____

   c. Limitations in my life such as _____
_____

6. In my career or work, my body hatred causes: _____
_____

   a. Feeling of _____
_____

   b. Actions such as _____
_____

   c. Limitations in my life such as _____
_____

7. (If applicable) With my children (or my desire to have children), my body hatred causes:

_____

_____

a. Feeling of _____

_____

b. Actions such as _____

_____

c. Limitations in my life such as _____

_____

8. Other ways in which my body hatred affects and limits my life:

_____

_____

a. Feeling of _____

_____

b. Actions such as _____

_____

c. Limitations in my life such as _____

_____

_____

If you were able to be honest with yourself in the above exercise, you may be more aware of how your perception of your body is causing suffering and how your body hatred limits your life—how it cuts you out of things you want to do or prevents you from achieving goals or dreams you may have for your life. Given the suffering caused by body hatred, the next step is to change how you feel about your body. When you feel differently about your body, you can begin to treat it differently.

Changing How You Feel About Your Body

At this point, if you are reading this book, at least a part of you is committed to being healthier in body, mind, and spirit. You may have originally started hating your body because you thought it would help you lose weight, but by now you must realize that that hasn't worked for you. Let's be clear. No amount of dieting, overexercising, or obsessing about food or your body will change what really needs to change: how you think about your body. When you relate to your body differently, your thoughts, feelings, and behavior will all change for the better.

Accepting the Importance of Your Thoughts

You may doubt that your words and thoughts about your body have any effect on your body or on your behaviors. But your body is a living organism made of energy. In elegant experiments done in Japan, when water was exposed to positive versus negative words, and then later frozen, the water exposed to expressions of love and gratitude or classical music, for example, formed incredibly beautiful crystals. The water molecules exposed to negative sentiment became poorly formed crystals or didn't form crystals at all. The author of these studies, Masaru Emoto (2011, xxvi), wrote: "Words are very likely to have an enormous impact on the water that composes as much as 70 percent of our body, and this impact will in no small way affect our bodies." (The beautiful photographs of water crystals are found in his book *The Hidden Messages of Water.*)

If you have a pet or young children, or if you are in any relationship with another living being, you know that your words affect them very strongly. Shout at your kids and you can bring them to tears. Saying something mean to your partner in anger can scar your relationship for a long time. If words matter in your relationships with other people, surely they matter in your relationship with your own body, too.

Harsh words can provoke emotions such as shame, fear, anger, or sadness. This is true whether we hear those words from other people or inflict them on ourselves. It's useful to be able to identify the emotions that lie beneath your beliefs and judgments about yourself. Say you believe that you're defective. "Defective" isn't an emotion; when you say that you "feel defective," what's really going on is that you feel *ashamed.*

So, what have your words and your thoughts been telling your body? Is this the message you want to give? How do you think the energy of your body is affected by your words? What emotions do your own words provoke in you? Is this the way you want to feel? These questions are not posed as another way to shame you. They are here to help you wake up to the reality that your body is listening to what you say and responding, just as it listens to what others have said about you. If you grew up in a home in which you didn't feel loved or respected, you may have decided that something was wrong with you. Sometimes that decision leads to another belief, that if you could just change the way you look, perhaps people—your parents, your peers, or others—would like you and then you'd get your needs met. If you think about this, it makes perfect sense that a child or a young adult may have drawn these conclusions and then set about making it happen. We all want and deserve love. Now that you are an adult, you may have realized that even though the child's point of view was valid, it no longer serves you as an adult. If you are willing, in the next exercise you can begin the process of letting go of these beliefs about your body that no longer work.

EXERCISE:
Clearing the Way for a Mature Relationship with Your Body

In the exercise below, take time to delve into how your current relationship with your body came about and what beliefs were formed from the past. This will prepare you to form a new relationship with your body—one that is more mature and more effective.

Thinking back to the earliest time you remember (or any earlier time you remember) feeling bad about your body:

See if you can remember the situation that may have caused you to feel bad about your body. (Example: *In Ariel's case, she remembered sitting in gym class with her two friends and comparing her thighs to theirs and feeling "gross."*)

_____

_____

_____

Identify the emotion you felt in this situation. (Example: *Since "gross" isn't an emotion, when Ariel was asked this question, she responded that she felt fear. She was afraid that no one would ever like her, and she remembered her mother telling her that she would never find a husband if she got any bigger.*)

_____

_____

_____

See if you can think of any decision you made in that moment or during other situations that formed a solution to your problem. (Example: *Ariel decided that she would make herself smaller. She knew she couldn't get shorter, so she focused on getting thinner so that she would not seem so huge and gross. This decision led to years of dieting and food addiction behaviors.*)

_____

_____

_____

Try to put yourself in your younger self's place and imagine what she needed in that situation. (Example: *Ariel had the insight that her younger self just needed some support and an understanding that she was not really huge. If she had understood that her early puberty is what caused her feelings and that eventually the other kids would catch up with her, this understanding would have helped. When she was older she spoke to an older cousin who, unbeknownst to her, had also had an early puberty but was a perfectly normal size now. Had she been able to talk with her about this, or had her mother been more supportive, it would have helped.*)

_____

_____

_____

_____

_____

Sometimes years of suffering can be caused by experiences that you were unable to understand or didn't know how to handle, or were too young to understand or cope with. It is important to realize that your brain and your body catalog all of the experiences you have. Whatever those experiences are or were—whether trauma, neglect, physical abuse, growing up in a household that emphasized the thin ideal, or growing up in a family in which your genetic makeup made you a different size than other members of the family—all of your past experiences have an impact on your body as well as on your mind and spirit. As you come to understand how your experiences have shaped your relationship with your body, you can begin to let go of beliefs that no longer serve you and "solutions" that don't really work.

Relating to Your Body in a New Way

In chapter 5, you made a start in changing your relationship with your body. This is your time now to decide how you want to relate to your body going forward. Do you want to continue to send your body negative messages, or would you like to experience a different way of relating? Can you imagine what it would be like if you stopped struggling against your body and started working with it, how different things might be? Let's explore this in the next exercise, which employs the concept of unconditional positive regard toward your body. Unconditional positive regard (http://en.wikipedia.org/wiki/Unconditional_positive_regard) is a concept developed by psychologist Carl Rogers that embodies a basic acceptance and support of a person no matter what that person says or does. Carl Rogers wrote that all people have within themselves vast resources for self-understanding and for changing their self-concept, attitudes, and behaviors if the right climate can be provided. You can apply the same approach to changing your relationship to your body. No matter how you feel your body has failed you, no matter what your thoughts tell you about your body, you can declare unconditional positive regard toward your body, thereby providing a nurturing climate for a new, more mature relationship with your body.

EXERCISE:
Imagining Your World Without Body Hatred

In the following exercise, make a list of statements of *unconditional positive regard* toward your body. I have listed a few possibilities to get you started. Then respond to the question below each statement. Even if your body-hatred thoughts continue to surface, see if you can connect with your heart and find enough compassion to list statements that represent your intention or desire for positive regard.

1. My body is wise. How is my body wise? (Example: *My body tells me when I'm tired even when I don't want to listen.*)

    _____

    _____

    If I were to act as if this were true, how would my thoughts about and behavior toward my body be different?

    _____

    _____

2. My body is strong. How is my body strong?

    _____

    _____

    If I were to act as if this were true, how would my thoughts about and behavior toward my body be different?

    _____

    _____

3. My body is worth taking care of. Why?

_____

_____

If I were to act as if this were true, how would my thoughts about and behavior toward my body be different?

_____

_____

4. I am content with my body. Why am I content?

_____

_____

If I were to act as if this were true, how would my thoughts about and behavior toward my body be different?

_____

_____

5. Other: _____

_____

If I were to act as if this were true, how would my thoughts about and behavior toward my body be different?

_____

_____

6. Other: _____

_____

If I were to act as if this were true, how would my thoughts about and behavior toward my body be different?

_____

_____

_____

Every living organism thrives better and is happier in a climate that nurtures its growth. Your body is no different. You can continue to use these statements of unconditional positive regard as affirmations by putting them in your smartphone as a "thought for the day," or journaling about them, or putting them on sticky notes and posting them around your house. It may sound like a silly thing to do, but this technique can help you shift your thoughts away from negative, self-defeating body hatred and begin to reinforce these more positive messages.

I hope that your answers to these questions have given you a glimpse of the new relationship you can develop with your body as you begin to regard yourself with love and compassion. After so many years of seeing your body as flawed, it may be challenging to shift to a more positive view. But with patience and commitment, it is entirely possible to learn to treat yourself more kindly.

EXERCISE:
Next Steps to Relating to Your Body in a Different Way

Now that you've begun to envision a more gentle, loving relationship with your own body, how do you move toward actually having this new relationship with yourself? The key is to take small steps.

Make a list of three things you feel you can do on a regular basis to practice positive regard toward your body. I've listed a few examples to get you started:

Get a regular haircut

Take a nap when I feel tired

Make a doctor's appointment to get a checkup

Wear jewelry to ornament and show off my body

Other: _____

Other: _____

Other: _____

Other: _____

_____

You may find yourself thinking that you don't deserve these things, or that they are self-indulgent. If this is the case, just remind yourself that you are inherently whole and worthy of care, simply because you're human. Would you ask your best friend to go without a haircut or a doctor's checkup? Would you tell your tired child he didn't deserve a nap? Why not extend the same care to yourself that you would naturally give to others? See if you can become more aware of thoughts of unworthiness, and when you do, imagine that these negative thoughts are written on a whiteboard and you are erasing them as quickly as the letters appear. If you do this visualization over and over, it will help you let go of thoughts of unworthiness and stay committed to steadily building a kinder, gentler relationship with the only body you'll ever have—the one you have right now.

Wrap-up

In a wonderful 2014 blog in the *Huffington Post*, Glennon Doyle Melton wrote, "Your body is not your masterpiece—your life is" (Melton 2014). She went on to say that, while we're told every day that our bodies are projects, it is really our life, our relationships, and our spiritual connection that should be our projects. Now more than ever, there are people in the media, writing blogs and posting videos, who are demonstrating that they love their bodies. There are women and men in larger bodies who are dancing their hearts out—doing ballet and hip hop or just moving their bodies to music. There are fat people who are pushing against the cultural norms and demonstrating how being healthy and happy in your body, no matter what its size, can free you up to live the life that you dream about and deserve.

Your body should not be a limit. You no longer have to buy into cultural norms or other people's ideals of what bodies should look like and do. These new models exist. Seek them out. When you change your perception and begin the process of accepting the beauty inherent in all bodies, including yours, you will be able to free up energy you've been using to obsess about your body to live life on your own terms. The next chapter will show you how to apply this new, more joyful and self-nurturing mindset to your relationship with food and eating.

CHAPTER 9

Savor Your Food, Heal Your Food Addiction

Carla was a thirty-nine-year-old woman, originally from Puerto Rico, who came to my office because she wanted to lose weight and get in better shape before her fortieth birthday. She was very vibrant, energetic, and talkative. She reported on the numerous diets she had been on in the past and how much weight she'd regained after each diet. She was now eating "only healthy and clean" foods and had begun weight lifting. She also drank protein shakes to boost muscle production. However, she hadn't lost as much weight as she'd expected and was afraid that she wouldn't be able to keep holding back on eating all her favorite foods— especially foods from her native Puerto Rico, such as beans and rice, fried plantains, and flan—for much longer. She felt that all of her native foods were "bad" foods and had stopped going to her mother's for Sunday dinner or eating in Puerto Rican restaurants in her neighborhood. Every time she thought about eating a beautiful coffee flan, she thought about how fat she felt and how much she hated her thighs. She had difficulty perceiving when she was physically hungry and when she was full. Her enjoyment of food had diminished significantly on her new diet, as she focused on losing weight. She wasn't sure she'd be able to lose the weight she wanted to lose and keep it off, and she wasn't sure she'd ever be able to enjoy food again.

In chapter 8, you learned about the relationship between food addiction and body image issues. While you can't insulate yourself entirely from cultural messages about what your body should look like, you can choose to be critical of those messages and form a new relationship with your body by making a conscious decision to treat it with kindness and respect. This chapter will focus on eating, and on how you can nurture your body with food.

You may be like many people with food addiction in that you divide food up into "good" foods and "bad" foods, just like Carla. You may deprive yourself of foods you think are bad for you and then end up craving them and overeating them at a later time. If you have obsessive thoughts about food, those thoughts may be related to how you use food to numb your feelings or deal with stress. It's also not uncommon, as discussed in previous chapters, to use food for comfort and pleasure. Perhaps you are like Carla, and your focus on food is all about fixing things you don't like about your body, rather than enjoying the food you are eating.

If you have any or all of these feelings about food, the next step in your recovery from food addiction is to shift from a focus on the number on the scale, or your body's size and shape, to a focus on nourishing your body and enjoying the experience of eating. This may seem like an impossible task, and you may feel lots of resistance to changing what you've been doing for so long. You may also feel that if you start letting yourself enjoy the food you eat, you'll gain more weight or binge even more. However, ask yourself whether what you've been doing is working. If it were working, it's doubtful you'd even be reading this book. I'm here to tell you that it is possible to truly nurture yourself by eating, and that you can learn to savor your food. Change is not easy, but it can begin with simple steps that you'll learn about in this chapter.

Attitudes and Beliefs About Food

As you've worked your way through this book, you have learned how food can take on many meanings in your life that have nothing to do with the food itself. People with food addiction are overly focused on food but often not aware of why. You've learned in earlier chapters some of the reasons why food can take on such a central and powerful role in your life—whether related to childhood trauma or neglect, food sensitivities, problems with emotional regulation, or trouble coping with stress. Hopefully this book has helped you identify some of these reasons and given you a higher level of awareness and better skills that you can now put into practice to help you change your relationship with food. In this chapter, you will be able to focus on your attitudes toward, and beliefs about, food and how those ideas fuel your food addiction. The exercise below will help get you started.

EXERCISE:
Ten Basic Food Principles

Let's start with ten basic principles. See how many of these statements you currently identify with. (Circle the number of the statements that resonate with you.)

1. Food is meant to nourish my body and also to be a source of pleasure.

2. I, like every other human in the world, need to eat to provide fuel for my body and my brain to function.

3. I deserve to eat foods that give me pleasure, not just foods that are part of a rigid diet for weight loss.

4. Food is neither good nor bad. Foods that are heavily processed or contain high quantities of sugar, fat, or salt—and thus are more likely to trigger my brain's reward mechanism—may be rightly considered "treats."

5. Treats aren't the only foods that are enjoyable to eat. Just about any foods that are cooked properly and seasoned well can be enjoyable to eat.

6. My body is an exquisitely tuned organism that knows how to manage its weight, and I don't need to restrict my food intake or constantly diet to make it work correctly.

7. Food should not be my only source of pleasure in life. If it is, it will take on too much power and control in my life. The solution is not to change the food or eating first. The solution is to invite more pleasure into my life.

8. I deserve to enjoy the food I eat bite by bite, moment by moment.

9. When I am paying attention to what I'm eating and how it makes my body feel, I know when I am hungry, what I am hungry for, and when I've eaten all that I need.

10. I no longer need to eat something for any reason other than it is a food I desire and enjoy, and it fuels my body.

Chances are you checked some but not all of the above statements. They are called basic principles because they describe underlying concepts that are sometimes hidden beneath the beliefs, fears, and obsessions associated with your food addiction. This chapter is about getting back to basics about food and relearning how to eat—with joy and with your awareness focused not on your emotions or on negative self-talk but on the food itself. You can help in this process by targeting one of the food principles each month and journaling about your experience. How easy (or difficult) is it for you to accept the truth of this principle? If you believed the principle was true, how would you approach food and eating? When you adjust your actions accordingly, what happens to your beliefs? This exploration will enable you to really make each principle meaningful from your own perspective, rather than forcing yourself to adopt a meaning that someone else developed. It is all right to modify the principles to make them fit your own evolving beliefs.

Food and Pleasure

As discussed in previous chapters, we live in a world that constantly encourages us to eat, drink, and snack. Your local mall probably has a food court, as most do, that offers a wide array of smells and tastes—many with foods that are high in sugar, salt, and fat that encourage your cravings and overwhelm your senses. Just smelling the aroma of cinnamon buns or buttered, sugared popcorn that seems to be piped into every level of the mall can make your mouth water and can be both your worst nightmare and, at the same time, your greatest fantasy. You may notice that these foods are very hard to resist, and you may find yourself eating a large meal without even thinking about it, when you only came to pick up your new cell phone or purchase a gift for your friend's birthday.

Food ads are another way you can get hooked into eating automatically, without thinking and without even being hungry—at least physically hungry. In the United States in 2013, the food and beverage industry spent over $136 million on advertising, and the restaurant industry spent over $6 billion dollars. McDonald's alone spent a total of $802 million on advertising. The nonalcoholic beverage industry (sodas, juice, and energy drinks) is no different, spending over $1 billion dollars worldwide in 2014. The incredible amount of money spent on advertising, especially ads targeting children, is believed to contribute to children's food preferences and negatively influence their weight and health. (The Rudd Center for Food Policy and Obesity N. D.; Statista, N. D.)

Given the monumental number of advertising dollars spent on food and beverages, can you really say you are choosing what to eat, or even when to eat? Can you say you eat what you eat for the joy of it, the taste of it, or the benefit of it? Or has your choice and enjoyment been hijacked by the savvy marketing people working for these big companies, who make you think that eating cinnamon buns every morning will make your life better, easier, or more fulfilling than eating oatmeal or another food that isn't like the crack cocaine of the food world?

Whenever I ask people with food addiction why they crave certain foods, they always say, "It's because I love to eat _____ ." But they don't always mean that they love the flavor or the experience of eating those foods. Rather, they mostly mean they love how the foods make them feel. For example, when I eat or even see strawberry shortcake, it takes me back to the feelings of happiness I felt around my grandmother. Food can bring us pleasure for many different reasons: there is the taste of the food itself, the enjoyment of eating with other people, and the pleasant memories that certain foods evoke, along with any associated emotions. In the exercise below, let's work together to identify which foods truly bring you pleasure and why.

EXERCISE:
Reclaiming the Joy of Eating

In the space below, write down one of the foods (or food fixes) you tend to obsess about, and then below that, write at least a paragraph describing why you find this food so pleasurable.

One of my food fixes is: _____

Here's why I love to eat this food: _____

_____

_____

_____

_____

_____

_____

_____

Below are some of the descriptive terms used by chefs, whose job it is to eat with attention and to describe the foods they love. Check off any of these descriptive words you used in your paragraph above:

- ☐ Savory
- ☐ Fruity
- ☐ Cold
- ☐ Warm
- ☐ Full-flavored
- ☐ Well-seasoned
- ☐ Sweet
- ☐ Depth of flavor

- ☐ Crunchy
- ☐ Creamy
- ☐ Juicy
- ☐ Spicy
- ☐ Rich
- ☐ Salty
- ☐ Fresh

If you find that you were unable to actually describe what you ate, you may be eating for reasons other than physical hunger. In the next section, you will be able to learn more about the different forms of hunger you may be feeding with your food fixes. Sometimes it's easy to confuse emotional hunger with physical hunger, so we'll look at physical hunger first.

Are You Really Hungry?

You may be like many people who've struggled with weight and with overeating—out of touch with your body. One of the most critical ways in which you disconnect from your body cues is by not being aware of when you are hungry and when you are full. Many people who binge eat are eating to the point of feeling sick because they are too full. Some people eat continuously throughout the day, so they never actually allow themselves to feel hungry. Others restrict their intake or don't eat all day, saving themselves for the big binge at night. In the next exercise, you can practice with the next several meals, identifying your level of hunger and fullness before and after you eat. This will help you get back in touch with the sensations related to physical hunger and satiety.

EXERCISE:
Learning to Know When You're Hungry

You should plan to do this exercise when you're ready to eat a meal. First, make sure you have an open space for your food. It's difficult to relax while eating if your table is filled with things you need to do or bills you need to pay. Don't eat in front of the television for this exercise, or at your desk or in your car.

Next, go through the levels of hunger and see if you can identify how hungry you are before eating.

1. **Starving:** You may have a headache, difficulty concentrating, dizziness, or lack of energy. These are symptoms you may have experienced while on a very restricted diet or when you skipped meals.

2. **Ravenous:** Your stomach is probably growling, and you may be cranky, irritable, or sick to your stomach.

3. **Hungry:** Your stomach feels empty, and you are thinking about food, but your hunger is not out of control.

4. **Full:** You feel satisfied. Your stomach is not overfull.

5. **Overfull:** You are starting to feel too full, and your stomach may feel slightly bloated.

6. **Maxed out:** You are uncomfortably full and may feel bloated and sluggish. You are not hungry at this point, so if you keep eating, it may be for emotional reasons.

7. **Thanksgiving Day:** You've gone too far. You are not hungry at all. You may feel sick to your stomach and sleepy from a food overload.

After you've finished eating, please go back through the hunger scale and identify how full you are or how hungry you still are. After each question below, describe what it feels like for you to be hungry or full. You can use your experience above or recall another time from the past.

1. When I am hungry, what I notice is: (Example from Carla: *My stomach feels empty, and it might be rumbling just a little.*)

   _____

   _____

2. When I am comfortably full, what I notice is: (Example from Carla: *I feel satisfied, with just a mild feeling of fullness in my stomach.*)

    _____

    _____

3. When I've eaten too much, what I notice is: (Example from Carla: *My stomach feels stretched, and I might feel a little sick.*)

    _____

    _____

4. The body sensation that I can reliably use to tell me when I should eat is: (Example from Carla: A *mild feeling of emptiness in my stomach.*)

    _____

5. The body sensation that I can reliably use to tell me when I am full and should stop eating is: (Example from Carla: A *mild feeling of fullness in my stomach.*)

    _____

    _____

Referring to the scale above, the best time to start eating is when you're between 2 and 3, and the best time to stop eating is between 3 and 4. If you find that you're eating when you are starving or ravenous, you will be more likely to overeat. If you're feeling this hungry, you should eat a small snack that you carry with you, so that when you sit down for your meal you'll be more in control. If you continue eating past number 4, you may be eating for emotional or stress-related reasons.

It's also important to let your body have enough time to feel full. If you tend to eat very fast, your body's hormones won't have enough time to sense fullness. Or if you eat all throughout the day, your body may not be able to give you hunger signals. For this reason, try to slow down your eating, and also eat regular meals during the day, rather than constantly snacking. Finally, it's crucial to ask yourself what you're feeling and whether you are physically or emotionally hungry. The next section will help you make this distinction.

What Are You Really Hungry For?

Beyond the physical sensations of hunger and fullness is the importance of making a distinction between physical hunger and emotional hunger. Physical hunger is thought to be related to contractions of the stomach muscles, or hunger pangs when severe. These contractions are triggered by the hormone ghrelin, which stimulates your desire to eat. Other hormones, such as leptin, have the opposite effect on appetite, making you feel full. If you've been overeating for some time, or if you tend to not pay attention to what you're eating or how your body feels, you may have gotten into the habit of eating when you are bored or stressed or angry. If so, you may have come to think of hunger not as a physical change in your body, but just as an "uncomfortable feeling." This kind of thinking can reinforce a pattern of eating when you're not physically hungry but want to use food to self-soothe or comfort yourself, or for its numbing effect. It's important to learn to distinguish what physical hunger feels like in your body. You can use the hunger scale above to work on that. In the next exercise, see if you can start making the distinction between physical hunger and emotional hunger.

EXERCISE:
Distinguishing Between Physical Hunger and Emotional Hunger

Answer the questions below to see if you can begin to separate out your physical from your emotional hunger.

1. What does it mean to be hungry? (Example: *For Carla, being hungry meant she was alone, without her family.*)

   _____

   _____

2. When you think you're hungry, ask yourself whether it is physical hunger or emotional hunger. Are you experiencing any of the physical hunger sensations you identified in the previous exercise? Are you experiencing an emotion that makes you want to eat?

   _____

3. What clues might reveal that you are eating for emotional reasons? (Example: *Carla noticed that when she was emotionally hungry she tended to crave more sweet foods and to eat very rapidly.*) Here's a list with examples to get you started:

I am more likely to eat certain foods when I'm eating from emotions.

I tend to eat in front of the television or at my desk, or just don't pay attention to what I'm eating.

Sometimes I've eaten a lot of something without even noticing.

_____

_____

_____

_____

4. Think of a time when you know you overate because of stress, boredom, or emotions. How did your body feel when you were overeating?

_____

_____

5. Based on your answers to these questions, what actions or behaviors would support you in continuing to be aware of when you're not physically hungry? (Example: *Carla found that if she wasn't sure if she was really hungry, she would eat a handful of almonds, yogurt, or another favorite snack. If she still felt hungry after that, she would eat more.*) Here is a list with some ideas to help you get started:

Plan to eat three meals a day and one snack so that you know your body is being nourished throughout the day.

Journal about your hunger and see if you are hungry around the same time of day, or in the same situations, and then plan to have a snack or do an activity at that time of day if you feel your hunger is more emotional than physical.

If you crave a certain food, for example, every afternoon, allow yourself to have a small portion of that food fix in a safe way. (Example: *Buy one cookie, not a whole box.*)

_____

_____

_____

_____

_____

_____

_____

Once you've gotten better at distinguishing between physical and emotional hunger, you're ready to focus more on learning, or relearning, to take pleasure in eating. Here's an exercise to help you get started.

_____

EXERCISE:
A Day of Joyful Eating

Imagine your favorite meals and describe them below. How would you go about finding or preparing these meals? And what other components would make them joyful for you?

1. My favorite breakfast

   a. The food I'd eat: (Example: *oatmeal, chai tea with soymilk*)

   _____

   _____

   _____

   _____

b. Who I'd eat with: (Example: *I love having breakfast with a good friend or with one of my sons or my granddaughter.*)

_____

_____

_____

c. How I would prepare or obtain these foods or where I'd go for breakfast: (Example: *I make this at home. I sometimes put frozen or fresh berries in it.*)

_____

_____

_____

2. My favorite lunch

a. The food I'd eat: (Example: *I love mini carnitas tacos! Depending on how hungry I am, I might get a side of rice and beans.*)

_____

_____

_____

b. Who I'd eat with: (Example: *Any friend who likes Mexican food, or by myself.*)

_____

_____

_____

c. How I would prepare or obtain these foods or where I'd go for lunch: (Example: *I have no idea how to cook carnitas, but I do know a great little dive near the beach where I can buy them.*)

_____

_____

_____

3. My favorite dinner

a. The food I'd eat: (Example: *I'd start with a really good salad, because I've recently realized I actually like salads if they are yummy. Then I'd have a lovely fish, like sea bass or salmon, along with roasted asparagus and roasted small potatoes. For dessert, I'd have one perfect dark chocolate truffle.*)

_____

_____

_____

b. Who I'd eat with: (Example: *Sometimes I like having dinner alone, and at other times I enjoy cooking and eating with friends.*)

_____

_____

_____

c. How I would prepare or obtain these foods or where I'd go for dinner: (Example: *There's a small market near me that always has fresh fish. I'd go to an organic grocery store for the salad and vegetables. For the chocolate, I'd go to a local place that's known for the best chocolates in the world!*)

_____

_____

_____

_____

Eating good food—in good company or alone—shopping and preparing food, and eating out are all ways to bring pleasure into your life. Breakfast should give you a happy send-off to your day and it should keep you going until lunch. Lunch should help sustain your focus and energy for the duration of your day. Dinner should be a satisfying conclusion to your day. It shouldn't keep you up at night or be too difficult to digest before bedtime. I invite you to use your journal to start writing about which foods you really like. Before each meal, ask yourself what you'd love to eat. Experiment with eating the foods you love and journal about how you feel when you do. Sometimes you'll find that the food you thought you'd love doesn't actually satisfy you. Maybe you ate something too heavy or too spicy. Write down what you observe and continue to eat foods you think you'll love. Don't feel obligated to clean your plate, especially if you find yourself eating something you really don't like.

Some people, as discussed in earlier chapters, may need to stay away from certain foods altogether. If that works for you, that's great. If it doesn't work for you and you find yourself restricting and then bingeing on foods you deprive yourself of, then try another way. This is your body and it is unique. For this reason, there is no one answer that fits everybody. Stay curious. Spend some time getting to know your own body, what it wants, and how it works. That's the best way to find out what works for you. In the next section, you'll find another tool that can help you practice eating for the right reasons.

Attentional Eating

You've probably heard of "mindful eating," a phrase that has been used to describe everything from being present while you're eating to gentle or silent meals and more. For the purpose of this book, I am using the phrase "attentional eating" which is more specific and easy to under-stand. When you pay attention to what you eat—how the food tastes and how it feels in your body—you can learn a lot of information about yourself as mentioned earlier. Learning about yourself should also include learning how to feed yourself in a way that brings you joy. Ask yourself how many meals you can remember that did this. I'm not talking about eating to get your "high" or telling yourself you love a food when, in fact, you really just crave it. I'm talking about the joy of eating with a group of people, or the joy of tasting certain foods and noticing how they feel in your mouth, how well prepared they are, and how they feel in your body.

While you may not rank every meal as the height of joy, you can aspire to having many or most of your meals be pleasant and enjoyable experiences. This is not something most people prioritize. If they did, they wouldn't be eating lunch at their desks while answering e-mails, or going through a drive-through and eating in their cars. Those ways of eating may be necessary from time to time, but it will amaze you when you begin to pay attention when you are eating, how much more pleasant it can be. The following is an exercise to help you begin to learn to eat with attention.

EXERCISE:
Attentional Eating

(adapted from Williams et al. 2007.)

For this exercise, you need a raisin or a small piece of any other fruit. You will also need to be in a quiet setting where you won't be disturbed.

Step 1—Observe: Put the raisin on a small plate on the table in front of you. Sit down and look at the raisin as if you are seeing it for the very first time. Take a few deep breaths to clear your mind. Notice its shape, its color, and the irregularities in its skin. Imagine how this one small raisin came to be. Imagine its transformation from a juicy grape to a dried raisin. Think about who might have picked those grapes, how the raisin made it to the place where you bought it, and all the people involved in growing this one tiny raisin.

Step 2—Touch: Now pick the raisin up and hold it in the palm of your hand. Notice its weight in your palm. Touch the raisin with your fingertips and notice what it feels like. *Notice, but do not buy into or grab onto, any thoughts that are coming up.*

Step 3—Smell: Hold the raisin up to your nose. Does it have a smell? How would you describe the smell? Does the smell make your mouth water? Is there any other body sensation that arises as you smell the raisin? *Notice, but do not pay attention to, any thoughts that are coming up.*

Step 4—Taste: Put the raisin on your tongue and hold it there. Without chewing it, notice how the raisin feels on your tongue. How would you describe the sensation on your tongue? Move the raisin around in your mouth and notice any sensations you feel.

Now you can start to slowly chew the raisin—very, very slowly. Pay attention to the taste as you bite into it. Is there a burst of flavor? Is there anything unexpected about the taste?

Notice, but do not pay attention to, any thoughts that are coming up.

Pause after you bite into the raisin, and again pay attention to the flavor, texture, and taste. Continue to chew, paying attention to any changes in the taste or texture.

Step 5—Swallow: After you have chewed the raisin enough and feel ready to swallow it, pay attention to your intention to swallow and then swallow. Notice whether you can feel the raisin moving from your mouth down into your esophagus and stomach. Imagine the journey it has taken just to nourish you. Express your gratitude toward this tiny raisin for its part in your journey to healing your relationship with food.

Attentional eating is part of what makes the experience of eating joyful. After all, you must notice your food in order to enjoy it. No matter what you are eating, if you eat with attention you will feel more satisfied and be less likely to overeat.

The famous Buddhist monk Thich Nhat Hanh suggests that "sharing a meal is not just to sustain our bodies and celebrate life's wonders, but also to experience freedom, joy, and the happiness of brotherhood and sisterhood, during the whole time of eating." He recommends starting meals with prayer or some form of contemplation, such as The Five Contemplations from Buddhist tradition (Nhat Hanh and Cheung 2010):

1. This food is a gift of the earth, the sky, numerous living beings, and much hard and loving work.

2. May we eat with mindfulness and gratitude so as to be worthy to receive this food.

3. May we recognize and transform our unwholesome mental formations, especially our greed, and learn to eat with moderation.

4. May we keep our compassion alive by eating in such a way that reduces the suffering of living beings, stops contributing to climate change, and heals and preserves our precious planet.

5. We accept this food so that we may nurture our brotherhood and sisterhood, strengthen our community, and nourish our ideal of serving all living beings.

The Five Contemplations give us a lot to aspire to. Whatever form of contemplation, prayer, or grace you choose, giving thanks for all that has been done to bring so much vibrant and nourishing food to your plate can give you a chance to get beyond your busy and worrisome thoughts, fears, and self-doubts and, through attentional eating, continue the process of healing from food addiction.

It's normal to hit some bumps along the road to recovery. A key piece of advice I give my clients is: if you give in to your cravings, do so with attention. Enjoy every morsel of the chocolate bar, every crumb of the cake or cookie you are eating. Avoid judging yourself for giving in to your cravings. Standing in judgment only makes you feel worse about yourself, which may lead you to overeat again. Be gentle with yourself. Remember, you're in the learning phase. You're like a toddler just learning to walk—and no one blames a toddler for falling down again and again. You shouldn't blame yourself either. If you eat with attention, you will be learning about yourself with each bite you take. In the long run, that's much more important in breaking an eating addiction than having a set of rigid rules, or trying to avoid foods you desire or obsess about.

Wrap-up

This chapter was all about helping you shift from obsessing about food to learning to truly savor your food. Eating is about nourishing our bodies, minds, and spirits. In this chapter, you've learned to notice what foods truly bring you pleasure, how to eat when you're hungry and stop when you're full, and to distinguish between physical and emotional hunger. Through attentional eating, you will be able, over time, to choose the foods that work best for your body. You will also be able to reduce the amount of mental energy you spend obsessing about food or your body. And hopefully, you will begin to experience the joy of eating well, without fear or shame or guilt.

In the next chapter, I'll discuss ways to build social and emotional support for your recovery. I'll also cover changes you can make to your environment to help you maintain your recovery. Finally, I'll help you write your own story of recovery. Writing this story is a way to create hope, and a pathway out of food addiction—a way to imagine your life without it.

CHAPTER 10

Taking Your Recovery to the Next Level

Joe is a thirty-nine-year-old man who has struggled with food addiction for many years. He has been to an inpatient treatment program, where I was his physician. At the time of his admission, his marriage was "on the rocks" and he was terrified of losing his relationship with his two young children. His wife was tired of his constant yo-yo dieting and his obsession with food and with his body. What I first noticed about Joe was that he was somewhat of a hipster: he thought of himself as having sophisticated tastes and preferences about food. Food was his drug of choice, but he repeatedly told me that his addictions were to healthy foods with only occasional forays into junk foods. He loved cooking and, in fact, owned a successful restaurant. But he found it very difficult to manage the stress associated with owning his own business and reported that this stress was a big trigger for his addiction.

Joe was also very sensitive to criticism, or the suggestion that his perceptions might in any way be flawed. For example, when I pointed out that his pattern was to run away from challenges rather than facing them head-on, he got very angry and abruptly left his therapy session. His inability to listen to constructive criticism initially hindered his ability to really understand his addiction. However, he was able to develop some relationships while in treatment, and over time learned to take feedback from his peers without getting angry. These relationships provided social support for him and helped him stay on track even after his discharge from the treatment program. So when he returned to his life, he had people he could turn to for support in staying on track—something he'd never had before. By the end of his stay in treatment, Joe had written a letter to me, apologizing for leaving our session so abruptly and also for some of the things he had said behind my back when he was angry. This was a very important sign of his spiritual growth through the process of treatment. As he stated in his letter, he realized that what he was lacking was compassion, especially for himself. In fact, he now had enough insight to recognize that his anger at me was really anger and judgments about himself. These insights signaled to me that Joe's mental well-being was improving at the same time as his physical well-being. He felt better physically because he was no longer obsessing about food and restricting and bingeing. He felt better mentally because he was able to see himself with compassion, listen to others without taking things personally, and be accountable for his mistakes. Having insights into who he was as a person and being able to accept himself (the good with the bad) will enable him to be stronger and not have the need to use food to deal with the normal ups and downs of life.

In the last chapter, you worked on changing how you experience and use food in your life. With food addiction, you may have spent most of your mental energy obsessing about food and about your body. As you recover and as your obsessions gradually become less prominent in your life, you will find that food begins to take its rightful place as a way to nourish and take care of your body, mind, and spirit. Instead of eating just to numb yourself, to satisfy cravings, or to deal with stress or your emotions, you may be learning to truly enjoy food and to be more curious about how food affects your body. In the process, you may find yourself wanting to explore other ways to find enjoyment in life. This desire may open you up to a whole new world of pleasurable experiences that, for whatever reason, you were not open to in the past.

Making lifestyle changes (what you eat, how active you are, how you manage stress) not only directly helps you overcome an eating addiction but can have long-lasting effects even on the genetic level. If you're like many individuals who have a food addiction, you may worry about how this disorder is affecting your children. Just know that working on your recovery as you are doing now will help reduce their risk for addictive and impulsive disorders in their lives. Perhaps you, like Joe, have come to realize that your addiction has put a strain on your interactions with other people. By nurturing yourself, healing yourself, you will have more space to be involved in your important relationships, and you'll find these other relationships to be more pleasurable than your relationship with food.

Taking Your Recovery to the Next Level

I am confident that your recovery from your eating addiction is proceeding at the rate it should. As you have been reading and working through this book, it is my hope that you've begun to see some obvious changes in your life. It takes time to make these changes, and you may be impatient thinking you haven't done enough or come far enough. I encourage you to give yourself credit for whatever changes, no matter how small, you've been able to make. In this chapter, you will explore ways to take your recovery to the next level by focusing on a few key areas that signal the strength and depth of your recovery. Remember the Five Levels of Healing and how this road map to recovery takes you deeper than just the superficial level of behaviors to more understanding of the things that drive your behaviors—such as emotions, core beliefs, and body sensations. The road map leads you to finding the deeper needs of your spirit or your soul. To find joy and peace, you have been learning how to go deeper, become more aware, and pay more attention to these different levels. This all takes you to creating a life in which you don't just survive, but thrive! Let's begin by talking about the importance of spirituality and social support.

Are You Getting Social Support?

Stress is a common cause of relapse in any addiction. While we all have stress, social support can mitigate the negative effects of stress. Social support involves interacting with others who can offer emotional concern and information and can help you see a different perspective on your problems. People with reward deficiency syndrome (RDS), as discussed in earlier chapters, may lack coping skills for dealing with stressful situations. (Laudet et al. 2006). For people with body dissatisfaction and a focus on body image issues, social support can be a protective factor and is associated with a lower risk for depression and substance use (Stice 2002). If you have a high level of social support, your eating addiction symptoms and body image issues are likely to be less problematic than they are for someone without social support. This means that social support can, in many ways, reduce the risks of other factors that are a part of food addiction. In fact, one study concluded that recovery from an eating disorder is mostly the result of connection to yourself and to others. In general, your social network provides the foundation for building a healthy identity and healthy emotional development, and for giving your life meaning (Leonidas and dos Santos 2014).

Social support can come from friends and family members, religious communities, colleagues or coworkers, or neighbors, and also from 12-Step communities. It can involve emotional support, sharing your story with others (called disclosure), gaining information, or seeking advice. Online forums, a newer method of obtaining support (Flynn and Stana 2012), can also be an effective component of a social network. Because you are early in your journey, it's very important that the new relationships you seek out don't follow old patterns. For this reason, here are a few words of caution to keep in mind while building your support network:

- Avoid repeatedly seeking support from people or places whose feedback is negative or demeaning, or makes you feel you are overly dependent.

- Be aware that not everyone with food addiction has done the type of in-depth recovery work you are doing. If others who have food addiction offer support, explore with them how long they have been in recovery and what they feel has helped them most. (Remember that a focus on weight loss, or on avoiding certain foods, can be the earliest form of recovery work.)

- Avoid people, places, or online sites that promote dieting or losing weight above all else, as these will only trigger your feelings of insecurity and may lead to a worsening of your food cravings and body image obsessions.

One of the most common ways people with addiction find social support is through a 12-Step community of people who are dealing with the same or similar problems. You can consider Food Addicts in Recovery Anonymous (http://www.foodaddicts.org) or Food Addicts

Anonymous (http://www.foodaddictsanonymous.org). These groups may also provide a deepening of your recovery work through the use of the 12 Steps of recovery from food addiction. The use of 12-Step groups can serve to provide structure for people with addictions who have often grown up without structure. The 12 Steps, themselves, provide a road map for what life is like in recovery. Many people with eating addictions are not familiar with these types of meetings and may feel too much shame and embarrassment to actually go to a meeting. My suggestion to overcoming any reluctance you have is to encourage you to take a friend you trust with you to a meeting, or try a phone or e-mail meeting first. These groups can be a very powerful form of social support, and if you are able to access this form of support, you, like many of my patients, may be surprised by how good it feels to not have to explain yourself to anyone because everyone at the meeting will understand what you're struggling with.

Another concern that people may have about 12-Step meetings is the "spiritual" component. You may not be religious or spiritual at all, but it is important for you to nourish your spirit in some way in order for your recovery to flourish. This subject will be discussed in general in the next section.

Are You Nourishing Your Spirit?

If you don't have any spiritual practices or haven't been raised in a spiritual or religious tradition, you may be skeptical about the need for nourishing your spirit. RDS researcher Kenneth Blum has written that spiritual connection actually increases the release of dopamine in your brain, which can help with the many symptoms of RDS—including cravings (Blum 2015). Other researchers have found that meditation combined with some type of spiritual belief or connection may promote dopamine release in the brain that could translate to a reduction in relapse risk (Brefczynski-Lewis et al 2007; Kozasa et al. 2012).

Nourishing your spirit may involve opening yourself up to a connection to nature or being close with a pet. Any experience that can promote a sense of awe—like watching a sunset or listening to the sounds of birds in nature or going to the symphony—is a way to nourish your spirit. Any expansion in your level of consciousness (sometimes called spiritual awakening) that improves your compassion for others and yourself strengthens your recovery. This is illustrated in Joe's story, by his insight about his interaction in our session and how this led to his recognition that compassion for himself and others would enable him to have deeper bonds in relationships, without the judgment and anger that came from taking things so personally. I'm sure you've felt this too, at some time in your life—for example, at the birth of a child or grandchild, or when you fell in love for the first time. It's hard to describe, but you know what it feels like—it's a connection to love, to awe, and to a new level of awareness. This is what leads to compassion.

The most important person to have compassion for is yourself. The deepest of the Five Levels of Healing (soul satisfaction) is awakening to who you truly are—seeing yourself, your flaws, and your mistakes with compassion. This is what happened for Joe, and this shift was a clear sign that he was moving beyond just the behavioral level of recovery. Over the time he was in treatment, as he came to know himself, stop judging his past, and accept his character flaws, he began to feel more compassion toward other people as well.

Many people who are in recovery from addictions stay at the superficial level, as in not drinking or not bingeing. While abstinence from behaviors is very important, it should be seen as the *gateway for a deeper understanding* of yourself and your addiction—not an end result. Deepening your recovery by awakening your spiritual connection or by nourishing your spirit brings with it more security in your recovery and a deeper sense of peace and joy in your life. As you connect with something greater than yourself (nature, God, awe, love), you will find yourself less focused on how you look and on the desire to binge or overeat. This connection could come through relationships and social support, but it should be something you can generate internally by finding activities and daily practices that foster this experience. Recovery cannot be based on the willpower that many people use to stop their behaviors. This is a shaky foundation. You build a stronger foundation when you go deeper into yourself, as described by the Five Levels. This is in fact what research shows. Awakening to knowing your true self is associated with lower rates of substance-seeking behaviors (Galanter et al. 2013). This means that spiritual awakening or nourishing your spirit is not for some abstract purpose, but actually can help your brain recover and lower your risk for relapsing. There are many ways to satisfy your soul's yearnings for fulfillment, connection, and a sense of meaning in life. Blum says it best: "Finding happiness may not only reside in our genome (your genetic makeup) but may indeed be impacted by positive meditative practices, positive psychology, spiritual acceptance, and taking inventory of ourselves—one day at a time" (Blum et al. 2015, 17).

Are You Prioritizing Your Own Well-Being?

One of the hallmarks of addiction is that the substance you see yourself addicted to is put above all else—whether that be food or alcohol or illicit drugs. You may feel like you're putting yourself first by obsessing about food or about your body, but actually you're either putting external appearance first or putting food used to satisfy cravings first. What would it look like to put your own well-being first?

PRIORITIZING YOUR PHYSICAL WELL-BEING

You may not have thought about what makes you feel good physically for a long time. From a medical standpoint, what the physical body needs to feel good includes energy or nourishment, some type of movement, and rest and relaxation. Think about how your body feels when you're stressed out and exhausted. Does your neck ache? Do you have heart palpitations? Do your muscles feel tight? These are examples of your body not feeling so good. Another example is how your body feels when you've skipped meals all day. Do you get a headache, or feel dizzy or light-headed? Do you feel tired or irritable? One of the important skills you will learn in recovery is to be more aware of what's going on in your body (and your mind). This awareness will enable you to make choices that will assist you in improving your physical well-being. Below are some ways in which you may begin to think about helping your body to feel its best.

Get enough rest. Lack of sleep is, by itself, associated with weight gain, emotional eating, and food cravings. Most people need seven to nine hours of sleep a night. No one can tell you how much you need, but if you pay attention to how you feel physically when you wake up in the morning, you will have a good idea of whether you've gotten enough sleep or not. You should consult your health care provider or ask for a referral to a sleep specialist if you continue having trouble falling or staying asleep, or if you don't feel refreshed when you wake up.

Nourish your body. You've learned a lot about eating in this book. What I'd like to point you toward now is what the future of eating in recovery may look like. This is based on my experience of working with people with eating disorders for extended periods of time and seeing how their eating behaviors change five or ten years into their recovery. Here are some of these observations:

- People who are well into recovery eat because they are hungry.

- Long-term recovered people eat foods they really love and foods that make them feel good. While you need to have some structure around what you eat when you're new in recovery, over time you will learn to listen to how the food you eat makes you feel.

- People in long-term recovery no longer choose what to eat based on calories, what makes them feel full, or whether a food is "good" or "bad." The physical body is an amazing feedback organism—if you are paying attention, you will learn how to work with, instead of against, your body's needs.

Move your body. Your body wants to be in motion, doing something it loves. You may or may not consider yourself an "athletic" person, so it is best to think not about exercising but just about being active. Can you walk to get your coffee in the morning rather than driving? When you're at work, can you take the stairs rather than the elevator? Beyond this, are there any forms of body movement that you may have been attracted to but talked yourself out of?—for example, martial arts or aerial silk workouts. (Look it up.) Did you used to like to swim as a kid, or ride a bicycle? Whatever moves you, whatever you feel attracted to, you should try. If you're worried about being self-conscious, you can try getting a friend to go with you or you can take an individual class first—whichever makes you feel more comfortable. The goal is just to sit less and move more.

Being healthy is about having a body that supports you in all that you choose to do. For this to happen, your body must have nutrients, must get enough rest, and must have some physical activity on a regular basis. It's not asking for much—just to be provided with a chance to show you how great it feels when you take care of yourself!

PRIORITIZING YOUR MENTAL WELL-BEING

Think of a time when your mind has not felt good—for example, when your mind was racing or worrying or full of anxious thoughts. You might have felt there was nothing you could do to change that. But there are several steps you can take to bring mental well-being to the forefront:

- **Try to quiet your mind,** whenever possible. Practices such as prayer, meditation, or any activity that takes your mind off your day-to-day problems can help. Sometimes just listening to music or dancing in your living room can allow your mind a little bit of rest.

- **Question your old beliefs.** Don't allow old beliefs that no longer fit you continue to run your life. Question whether or not the things you believe to be absolute truths really are true at this point in your life. Also question negative thoughts such as *I'm so fat I'll never have...* (fill in the blank). See if you can challenge this kind of thinking instead of letting this old record continue to play over and over again, ruining your dreams for your future in recovery.

- **Stay conscious.** Another component of mental well-being is being able to catch yourself when you have slipped back into unconscious obsessive thoughts or behaviors. Being immersed in a habitual, negative frame of mind always promotes your food addiction thinking and behaviors. By becoming more aware, you can choose to think and act differently. This is about changing your way of being. With food addiction, you may have used food unconsciously—in other words, you may have found yourself with an empty box of donuts without any memory of reaching for the box. You also may have been unconscious about the emotions you were feeling, or the situations in your life you were responding to with food. When you stay conscious, you stay aware of what you are feeling, and aware of your desire to use food to numb it or "go unconscious." When you stay conscious, you have more power to make the choices that support your recovery, instead of just acting unconsciously through food. When you feel confused or frustrated about anything, take that as a sign to stop and take a look at what you're about to do or say.

- **Don't take your thoughts too seriously.** The thoughts that run through your mind automatically and repetitively are probably not as meaningful and important as they seem. I'm not talking about the use of your mind to balance your checkbook or make important decisions. I am referring to the thoughts that constantly trip you up, make you fearful and anxious, or insert themselves into places where they don't belong. You can change your perception of these thoughts. You may be someone who believes that what your mind tells you is very important. Usually it isn't. With conscious awareness, you can learn to recognize these thoughts for what they are: the chatter of your mind. While you can't get rid of such thoughts, you can certainly practice paying them less attention. Think of them as junk mail. Just delete and move back into the active e-mail box.

Are You Prepared for Lapses?

You may be afraid to think about the possibility of slipping up in the future. In fact, many people believe that even talking about lapses gives you an excuse to go back to your old behaviors. The truth is that your cravings may come back when you least expect them. Maybe you'll be doing well, but then you get a promotion at work and have old feelings of insecurity come up. Next thing you know, you're standing at the refrigerator with an empty carton of ice cream in your hand. Or you may start up a new relationship and find that you're struggling with body shame or body hatred. Just remember, when your old thoughts, feelings, obsessions, or cravings return, that's no reason to despair. Most of my patients think, for some reason, that life is supposed to be perfect in recovery. This is a common fallacy. Somehow we forget that life is just life. It has its ups and downs. It's never been perfect and it won't be perfect in recovery. This is a fact that is best accepted early on. When feeling frustrated about having cravings, in the past you may have been able to assume they were all part of your eating addiction. Now, however, it's important for you to listen and learn from your body what cravings or other feelings might mean. Here are some things to keep in mind:

- **Don't make any assumptions.** Treat each "lapse" as a question mark: Have I really lapsed or am I experiencing a normal bodily reaction? Remember, your body will be learning and adjusting to all the changes you're making at the same time your mind is. Maybe you're having a craving because you just worked out for an hour, or because you haven't eaten since breakfast and it's now 6:00 p.m. The only way to distinguish these absolutely normal experiences of hunger from addictive cravings is to be observant. Stay curious about how your body works and remember that your body is always sending you messages. It's up to you to listen. Keep a journal of activities and hunger, and over time you will be able to see the patterns. In the beginning, you can try just eating a snack to see if your "cravings" are from hunger or from your eating addiction. If you get hungry every time you work out, then you should recognize this pattern and be ready to address that hunger.

- **Is it a lapse or an adjustment?** Sometimes you will have a lapse, but at other times, what you may have assumed is a lapse is just an adjustment. You'll have to redefine what a mistake or lapse is, versus what is just a sign that your body, mind, and spirit are making adjustments, adapting to new experiences, or providing information about the changes you are making. This is a normal part of your recovery. You will be making adjustments all the time. You don't have to judge yourself or be ashamed when something needs to change. Recovery from food addiction should include a hefty portion of reflection and questioning whether the meaning you've given to certain signs still fits. If you are craving sweets, is that a sign of a lapse, or are you just hungry? If you have a binge, is it because you waited too long to eat dinner, or is it a lapse? These are individual reflections that you will become better and better at doing if you stay aware of what you are feeling and don't get overly upset, even if you do decide you've lapsed. The most important predictor of long-term success is how long it takes you to recover from a lapse!

- **Don't judge yourself or allow others to judge you.** With each "mistake" you make, you have the opportunity to learn something about yourself, your body, your beliefs, or your thoughts. There is no perfect way to heal. In fact, wanting your recovery to be perfect comes from the same thoughts and beliefs that promote eating addiction. So allow yourself this time to make what you call mistakes, which I call learning experiences.

One important key to dealing with change is to stay flexible. You need to cultivate physical flexibility by doing stretches or other flexibility exercises. Similarly, you need to promote mental flexibility so that you don't become rigid in your thinking or overly attached to your beliefs. Part of mental flexibility is allowing yourself to make mistakes or have lapses without judging yourself too harshly. And when you stay flexible in spirit, you can continue growing as a person. All of these are important in long-term recovery.

I've summed up for you throughout this book the steps that are important to take to identify and become more aware of the causes of eating addiction and ways to recover. By this time, you are hopefully continuing to grow in your recovery. As part of taking your recovery to the next level, you may want to use the next exercise to write your own story of recovery.

EXERCISE:
Your Story of Recovery

Use this exercise to document the challenges and triumphs you've experienced on your journey from eating addiction. This will serve as a reminder for you of where you were perhaps even before you picked up this book, so that years from now when you've forgotten about how far you've come, you can be reminded of your achievements. I would encourage you to write as much as you remember in response to each prompt:

Document as much as you can remember about how childhood events contributed to your food addiction.

_____

_____

_____

_____

_____

Write about touchstones along the way in your addiction (for example, how you first became aware that you had a problem, how you sought help, and who has supported you along the way).

_____

_____

_____

_____

_____

Make a list of all the areas of your life that have been affected by your eating addiction.

_____

_____

_____

_____

_____

Think about times you struggled more than others and why.

_____

_____

_____

_____

_____

Ask yourself, and include in your story, significant insights you've had about yourself on your journey to recovery.

_____

_____

_____

_____

Make a list of the changes you've made so far—no matter how small or tenuous they may seem.

_____

_____

_____

_____

_____

_____

_____

Most importantly, imagine a future you, living life without food addiction.

_____

_____

_____

_____

_____

_____

_____

Put anything else in your story that seems important to you. Remember, it's *your* story, so you can personalize it in any way you see fit.

_____

_____

_____

_____

_____

_____

_____

_____

_____

_____

_____

_____

_____

_____

_____

_____

Wrap-up

You've done it! You've spent time and energy on yourself. You've learned about food addiction and about the many possible causes and contributing factors. You've learned about the importance of being more aware of your emotions and body sensations. You are on your way. While I haven't been able to speak to you in person, I feel as if I know you well and it is my hope for you, as my reader, that this book has helped you find space to create the life you so deserve. As your mind clears, your body strengthens, and your spirit begins to soar, you have so much happiness that awaits you. Please claim it for yourself. After all, you've worked hard for it, and it belongs to you!

References

Adam, T. C., and E. S. Epel. 2007. "Stress, Eating, and the Reward System." *Physiology and Behavior* 91: 449–458.

American Institute of Stress. N.D. "What Is Stress?" http://www.stress.org/what-is-stress/. Accessed March 16, 2017.

American Psychological Association. 2014. "More Sleep Would Make Most Americans Happier, Healthier and Safer." http://www.apa.org/research/action/sleep-deprivation.aspx. Accessed March 16, 2017.

Arrieta, M. C., L. Bistritz, and J. B. Meddings. 2006. "Alterations in Intestinal Permeability." *Gut* 10: 1512–1520.

Avena, N. M., P. Rada, and B. G. Hoebel. 2009. "Sugar and Fat Binging Have Notable Differences in Addictive-Like Behavior." *Journal of Nutrition* 139: 623–628.

Baillie-Hamilton, P. F. 2002. "Chemical Toxins: A Hypothesis to Explain the Global Obesity Epidemic." *Journal of Alternative and Complementary Medicine* 8: 185–192.

Bardo, M. T., R. L. Donohew, and N. G. Harrington. 1996. "Psychobiology of Novelty Seeking and Drug Seeking Behavior." *Behavioural Brain Research* 77: 23–43.

Bassareo, V., G. Di Chiara. 1997. "Differential Influence of Associative and Nonassociative Learning Mechanisms on the Responsiveness of Prefrontal and Accumbal Dopamine Transmission to Food Stimuli in Rats Fed *Ad Libitum*." *Journal of Neuroscience* 17: 851–861.

Bayol, S. A, B. H. Simbi, R. C. Fowkes, and N. C. Stickland. 2010. "A Maternal 'Junk Food' Diet in Pregnancy and Lactation Promotes Nonalcoholic Fatty Liver Disease in Rat Offspring." *Endocrinology* 151: 1451–1461.

Bearman, S. K., E. Martinez, E. Stice, and K. Presnell. 2006. "The Skinny on Body Dissatisfaction: A Longitudinal Study of Adolescent Girls and Boys." *Journal of Youth and Adolescence* 35: 217–229.

Behnke, M, V. C. Smith, Committee on Substance Abuse, and Committee on Fetus and Newborn. 2013. "Prenatal Substance Abuse: Short- and Long-Term Effects on the Exposed Fetus." *Pediatrics* 131: e1009–e1024.

Bello, N. T., and A. Hajnal. 2010. "Dopamine and Binge Eating Behaviors." *Pharmacology Biochemistry and Behavior* 97: 25–33.

Bergmeier, H., H. Skouteris, and M. Hetherington. 2015. "Systematic Research Review of Observational Approaches Used to Evaluate Mother-Child Mealtimes During Preschool Years." *American Journal of Clinical Nutrition* 101(7):7–15.

Berlin, H. A., and E. Hollander. 2008. "Understanding the Differences Between Impulsivity and Compulsivity." *Psychiatric Times*. http://www.psychiatrictimes.com/articles/under standing-differences-between-impulsivity-and-compulsivity. Accessed March 16, 2017.

Birbeck, D., and M. Drummond. 2006. "Young Children's Body Image: Bodies and Minds Under Construction." *International Education Journal* 7: 423–434.

Bischoff, S. C. 2011. "'Gut Health': A New Objective in Medicine?" *BMC Medicine* 9:24.

Blackledge, J. T., and S. C. Hayes. 2001. "Emotion Regulation in Acceptance and Commitment Therapy." *Journal of Clinical Psychology* 57: 243–255.

Block, J. P., Y. He, A. M. Zaslavsky, L. Ding, and J. Z. Ayanian. 2009. "Psychosocial Stress and Change in Weight Among US Adults." *American Journal of Epidemiology* 170: 181–192.

Blum, K., J. G. Cull, E. R. Braverman, and D. E. Comings. 1996. "Reward Deficiency Syndrome." *American Scientist* 84: 132–145.

Blum, K., E. R. Braverman, J. M. Holder, J. O. Lubar, V. J. Monastra, D. Miller, T. J. H. Chen and D. E. Comings. 2000. "The Reward Deficiency Syndrome: A Biogenetic Model for the Diagnosis and Treatment of Impulsive, Addictive, and Compulsive Behaviors." *Journal of Psychoactive Drugs* 32 Suppl: i–iv, 1–112.

Blum, K., A. L. C. Chen, M. Oscar-Berman, et al. 2011. "Generational Association Studies of Dopaminergic Genes in Reward Deficiency Syndrome (RDS) Subjects: Selecting Appropriate Phenotypes for Reward Dependence Behaviors." *International Journal of Environmental Research and Public Health* 8: 4425–4459.

Blum, K., J. Bailey, A. M. Gonzalez, M. Oscar-Berman, J. Liu, J. Giordano, E. Braverman, and M. Gold. 2011. "Neuro-genetics of Reward Deficiency Syndrome (RDS) as the Root Cause of 'Addiction Transfer': A New Phenomenon Common After Bariatric Surgery." *Journal of Genetic Syndromes and Gene Therapy* 2012(1): pii: S2–001.

Blum, K., B. Thompson, M. Oscar-Berman, J. Giordano, E. Braverman, J. Femino, D. Barh, W. Downs, T. Simpatico, and S. Schoelenthaler. 2013. "Genospirituality: Our Beliefs, Our Genomes, and Addictions." *Journal of Addiction Research and Therapy* 5: pii: 162.

Blum, K., M. Oscar-Berman, Z. Demetrovics, D. Barh, and M. S. Gold. 2014. "Genetic Addiction Risk Score (GARS): Molecular Neurogenetic Evidence for Predisposition to Reward Deficiency Syndrome (RDS)." *Molecular Neurobiology* 50: 765–796.

Blum, K., B. Thompson, D. Zsolt, J. Femino, J. Giordano, M. Oscar-Berman, S. Tietelbaum, D. E. Smith, A. K. Roy, G. Agan, J. Fratantonio, R. D. Badgaiyan, and M. S. Gold. 2015. "The Molecular Neurobiology of Twelve Step Programs and Fellowship: Connecting the Dots for Recovery." *Journal of Reward Deficiency Syndrome* 1: 46–64.

Bolton, M. A., I. Lobben and T. A. Stern. 2010. "The Impact of Body Image on Patient Care." *Primary Care Companion to the Journal of Clinical Psychiatry* 12: PCC.10r00947.

Brefczynski-Lewis, J. A., A. Lutz, H. S. Schaefer, D. B. Levinson and R. J. Davidson. 2007. "Neural Correlates of Attentional Expertise in Long-Term Meditation Practitioners." *Proceedings of the National Academy of Sciences of the United States of America* 104: 11483–11488.

Burmeister, J. M., N, Hinman, A. Koball, D. A. Hoffmann, and R. A. Carels. 2013. "Food Addiction in Adults Seeking Weight Loss Treatment. Implications for Psychosocial Health and Weight Loss." *Appetite* 60: 103–110.

Camilleri, M., K. Madsen, R. Spiller, B. Greenwood-Van Meerveld, and G. N. Verne. 2012. "Intestinal Barrier Function in Health and Gastrointestinal Disease." *Neurogastroenterology and Motility* 24: 503–512.

Cardinal, R. N., C. A. Winstanley, T. W. Robbins, and B. J. Everitt. 2004. "Limbic Corticostriatal Systems and Delayed Reinforcement." *Annals of the New York Academy of Sciences* 1021: 33–50.

Cash, T. F., J. Thériault, and N. M. Annis. 2004. "Body Image in an Interpersonal Context: Adult Attachment, Fear of Intimacy, and Social Anxiety." *Journal of Social and Clinical Psychology* 23: 89–103.

Cassidy, J., and J. J. Mohr. 2001. "Unsolvable Fear, Trauma, and Psychopathology: Theory, Research, and Clinical Considerations Related to Disorganized Attachment Across the Life Span." *Clinical Psychology: Science and Practice* 8: 275–298.

Childs, E., and H. de Wit. 2014. "Regular Exercise Is Associated with Emotional Resilience to Acute Stress in Healthy Adults." *Frontiers in Physiology* 5: 161.

Chua, J. L., S. Touyz, and A. J. Hill. 2004. "Negative Mood-Induced Overeating in Obese Binge Eaters: An Experimental Study." *International Journal of Obesity and Related Metabolic Disorders* 28: 606–610.

Corstorphine, E., V. Mountford, S. Tomlinson, G. Waller, and C. Meyer. 2007. "Distress Tolerance in the Eating Disorders." *Eating Behaviors* 8: 91–97.

Crawford, M., and O. U. Cadogan. 2008. *Nutrition and Mental Health: A Handbook.* East Sussex, UK: Pavilion Publishing and Media.

Crinnion, W. J. 2000. "Environmental Medicine, Part 1: The Human Burden of Environmental Toxins and Their Common Health Effects." *Alternative Medicine Review* 5: 52–63.

Cummings, J. A., L. G, Clemens, and A. A. Nunez. 2010. "Mother Counts: How Effects of Environmental Contaminants on Maternal Care Could Affect the Offspring and Future Generations." *Frontiers in Neuroendocrinology* 31: 440–451.

Dallman, M. F. 2010. "Stress-Induced Obesity and the Emotional Nervous System." *Trends in Endocrinology and Metabolism* 21: 159–165.

Dallman, M. F., N. C. Pecoraro, and S. E. la Fleur. 2005. "Chronic Stress and Comfort Foods: Self-Medication and Abdominal Obesity." *Brain, Behavior, and Immunity* 19: 275–280.

Davis, P. 2008. Oprah & Eckhart Tolle – A New Earth, Feeding the Body with Spiritual Energy & Overcoming Obesity. August 7. http://mexpjscike.blogspot.com/2008/08/oprah -eckhart-tolle-new-earth-feeding.html. Accessed March 16, 2017.

Deng, Y., B. Misselwitz, N. Dai, and M. Fox. 2015. "Lactose Intolerance in Adults: Biological Mechanism and Dietary Management." *Nutrients* 7: 8020–8035.

Depue, R. A., and P. F. Collins. 1999. "Neurobiology of the Structure of Personality: Dopamine, Facilitation of Incentive Motivation, and Extraversion." *Behavioral and Brain Sciences* 22: 491–517.

Elfhag, K., and S. Rössner. 2005. "Who Succeeds in Maintaining Weight Loss? A Conceptual Review of Factors Associated with Weight Loss Maintenance and Weight Regain." *Obesity Review* 6: 67–85.

Emoto, M. 2011. *The Hidden Messages in Water.* New York: Simon & Schuster.

Enoch, M. A. 2011. "The Role of Early Life Stress as a Predictor for Alcohol and Drug Dependence." *Psychopharmacology (Berlin)* 214: 17–31.

Felitti, V. J., R. F. Anda, D. Nordenberg, D. F. Williamson, A. M. Spitz, V. Edwards, M. D. Koss, and J. S. Marks. 1998. "Relationship of Childhood Abuse and Household Dysfunction to Many of the Leading Causes of Death in Adults. The Adverse Childhood Experiences (ACE) Study." *American Journal of Preventive Medicine* 14: 245–258.

Field, A. E., K. R. Sonneville, R. D. Crosby, S. A. Swanson, K. T. Eddy, C. A. Camargo Jr., N. J Horton, and N. Micali. 2014. "Prospective Associations of Concerns About Physique and the Development of Obesity, Binge Drinking, and Drug Use Among Adolescent Boys and Young Adult Men." *Journal of the American Medical Association Pediatrics* 168: 34–39.

Flynn, M. A., and A. Stana. 2012. "Social Support in a Men's Online Eating Disorder Forum." *International Journal of Men's Health* 11: 150–169.

Franz, M. J., J. J. VanWormer, A. L. Crain, J. L. Boucher, T. Histon, W. Caplan, J. D. Bowman, and N. P. Pronk. 2007. "Weight-Loss Outcomes: A Systematic Review and Meta-analysis of Weight-Loss Clinical Trials with a Minimum 1-Year Follow-up." *Journal of the American Dietetic Association* 107: 1755–1767.

Freud, S. 1938. *An Outline of Psychoanalysis.* London: Hogarth; p. 188.

Fullerton, D. T., C. Getto, W. J. Swift, and I. H. Carlson. 1985. "Sugar, Opioids, and Binge Eating." *Brain Research Bulletin* 14: 673–680.

Galanter, M., H. Dermatis, S. Post, and C. Sampson. 2013. "Spirituality-Based Recovery from Drug Addiction in the Twelve-Step Fellowship of Narcotics Anonymous." *Journal of Addiction Medicine* 7: 189–195.

Gearhardt, A. N., W. R. Corbin, and K. D. Brownell. 2009. "Preliminary Validation of the Yale Food Addiction Scale." *Appetite* 52: 430–436.

Gearhardt, A. N., M. A. White, and M. N. Potenza. 2011a. "Binge Eating Disorder and Food Addiction." *Current Drug Abuse Reviews* 4: 201–207.

Gearhardt, A. N., S. Yokum, P. T. Orr, E. Stice, W. R. Corbin, and K. D. Brownell. 2011b. "Neural Correlates of Food Addiction." *Archives of General Psychiatry* 68: 808–816.

Gluck, M. E, A. Geliebter, J. Hung, and E. Yahav. 2004. "Cortisol, Hunger, and Desire to Binge Eat Following a Cold Stress Test in Obese Women with Binge Eating Disorder." *Psychosomatic Medicine* 66: 876–881.

Grandjean, P., D. Bellinger, A. Bergman, S. Cordier, G. Davey-Smith, B. Eskenzi, et al. 2008. "The Faroes Statement: Human Health Effect of Developmental Exposure to Chemicals in Our Environment." *Basic and Clinical Pharmacology and Toxicology* 102: 73–75.

Greeno, C. G., and R. R. Wing. 1994. "Stress-Induced Eating." *Psychological Bulletin* 115: 444–464.

Hammons, A. J., and B. H. Fiese. 2011. "Is Frequency of Shared Meals Related to the Nutritional Health of Children and Adolescents?" *Pediatrics* 127: e1565-e1574.

Hanson, R. F., and E. G. Spratt. 2000. "Reactive Attachment Disorder: What We Know About the Disorder and Implications for Treatment." *Child Maltreatment* 5: 137–145.

Hays, N. P., and S. B. Roberts. 2008. "Aspects of Eating Behaviors 'Disinhibition' and 'Restraint' Are Related to Weight Gain and BMI in Women." *Obesity (Silver Spring)* 16: 52–58.

Hellemans, K. G. C., J. H. Sliwowska, P. Verma, and J. Weinberg. 2010. "Prenatal Alcohol Exposure: Fetal Programming and Later Life Vulnerability to Stress, Depression and Anxiety Disorders." *Neuroscience and Biobehavioral Reviews* 34: 791–807.

Hernandez, L., and B. G. Hoebel. 1988. "Food Reward and Cocaine Increase Extracellular Dopamine in the Nucleus Accumbens as Measured by Microdialysis." *Life Sciences* 42: 1705–1712.

Holford, P. 2003. *Optimum Nutrition for the Mind.* London: Piatkus.

Huang X. F., K. Zavitsanou, X. Huang, Y. Yu, H. Wang, F. Chen, A. J. Lawrence, and C. Deng. 2006. "Dopamine Transporter and D2 Receptor Binding Densities in Mice Prone or Resistant to Chronic High Fat Diet-Induced Obesity." *Behavioral Brain Research* 175: 415–419.

Hyman, M. A. 2010. "Environmental Toxins, Obesity, and Diabetes: An Emerging Risk Factor." *Alternative Therapies in Health and Medicine* 16: 56–58.

Ikemoto, S., and J. Panksepp. 1999. "The Relationship Between Self-Stimulation and Sniffing in Rats: Does a Common Brain System Mediate These Behaviors?" *Behavioural Brain Research* 61: 143.

Insel, T. R., and L. J. Young. 2001. "The Neurobiology of Attachment." *Nature Reviews Neuroscience* 2: 129–136.

Johnson, P. M., and P. J. Kenny. 2010. "Dopamine D2 Receptors in Addiction-Like Reward Dysfunction and Compulsive Eating in Obese Rats." *Nature Neuroscience* 13: 635–641.

Koob, G. F. 2009. "Neurobiological Substrates for the Dark Side of Compulsivity in Addiction." *Neuropharmacology* 56(Suppl 1): 18–31.

Koob, G. F., and M. Le Moal. 1997. "Drug Abuse: Hedonic Homeostatic Dysregulation." *Science* 278: 52–58.

Kozasa, E. H., J. R. Sato, S. S. Lacerda, M. A. Barreiros, J. Radvany, T. A. Russell, L. G. Sanches, L. E. Mello, and E. Amaro, Jr. 2012. "Meditation Training Increases Brain Efficiency in an Attention Task." *NeuroImage* 59: 745–749.

Kuiper, N. A., and N. McHale. 2009. "Humor Styles as Mediators Between Self-evaluative Standards and Psychological Well-being." *Journal of Psychology* 143: 359–376.

Laudet, A. B., K. Morgen, and W. L. White. 2006. "The Role of Social Supports, Spirituality, Religiousness, Life Meaning and Affiliation with 12-Step Fellowships in Quality of Life Satisfaction Among Individuals in Recovery from Alcohol and Drug Problems." *Alcoholism Treatment Quarterly* 24: 33–73.

Leonidas, C., and M. A. Dos Santos. 2014. "Social Support Networks and Eating Disorders: An Integrative Review of the Literature." *Neuropsychiatric Disease and Treatment* 10: 915–927.

Lima, A. A., A. M. Soares, N. L. Lima, R. M. Mota, B. L. Maciel, M. P. Kvalsund, L. J. Barrett, R. P. Fitzgerald, W. S. Blaner, and R. L. Guerrant. 2010. "Effects of Vitamin A Supplementation on Intestinal Barrier Function, Growth, Total Parasitic, and Specific *Giardia spp* Infections in Brazilian Children: A Prospective Randomized, Double-Blind, Placebo-Controlled Trial." *Journal of Pediatric Gastroenterology and Nutrition* 50: 309–315.

Madowitz, J., B. E. Matheson, and J. Liang. 2015. "The Relationship Between Eating Disorders and Sexual Trauma." *Eating and Weight Disorders* 20: 281–293.

Maida, A., A. Zota, K. A. Sjøberg, J. Schumacher, T. P. Sijmonsma, A. Pfenninger, et al. 2016. "A Liver Stress-Endocrine Nexus Promotes Metabolic Integrity During Dietary Protein Dilution." *Journal of Clinical Investigation* 126: 3263–3278.

Martinac, M., D. Pehar, D. Karlovic, D. Babic, D. Marcinko, and M. Jakovljevic. 2014. "Metabolic Syndrome, Activity of the Hypothalamic-Pituitary-Adrenal Axis, and Inflammatory Mediators in Depressive Disorder." *Acta Clinica Croatia* 53: 55–71.

Martin-Soelch, C., J. Linthicum, and M. Ernst. 2007. "Appetitive Conditioning: Neural Bases and Implications for Psychopathology." *Neuroscience and Biobehavioral Reviews* 31: 426–440.

McEwen, B. S. 2007. "Physiology and Neurobiology of Stress and Adaptation: Central Role of the Brain." *Physiological Reviews* 87: 873–904.

McKay, M., and P. Rogers. 2000. *The Anger Control Workbook.* Oakland, CA: New Harbinger Publications.

McKinley, N. M., and L. A. Randa. 2005. "Adult Attachment and Body Satisfaction. An Exploration of General and Specific Relationship Differences." *Body Image* 2: 209–218.

Melton, G. D. 2014. "Your Body Is Not Your Masterpiece." *The Huffington Post.* http://www .huffingtonpost.com/glennon-melton/your-body-is-not-your-masterpiece_b_5586341.html. Accessed March 16, 2017.

Meule A., and A. N. Gearhardt. 2014. "Five Years of the Yale Food Addiction Scale: Taking Stock and Moving Forward." *Current Addiction Reports* 1: 193–205.

Myers, A., and J. C. Rosen. 1999. "Obesity Stigmatization and Coping: Relation to Mental Health Symptoms, Body Image, and Self-esteem." *International Journal of Obesity and Related Metabolic Disorders* 23: 221–230.

Nadeau, K. 2011. "New Treatment May Desensitize Kids with Milk Allergies, Say Researchers." https://med.stanford.edu/news/all-news/2011/03/new-treatment-may-desensitize-kids-with -milk-allergies-say-researchers.html. Accessed February 3, 2017.

National Institute of Diabetes and Digestive and Kidney Diseases. 2016. "Celiac Disease." http://www.celiac.nih.gov/PDF/CeliacDiseaseChart_508.pdf. Accessed March 16, 2017.

National Institute on Drug Abuse. 2016. "The Science of Drug Abuse and Addiction: The Basics." http://www.drugabuse.gov/publications/media-guide/science-drug-abuse-addiction -basics. Accessed March 16, 2017.

Nelson, M., and J. Ogden. 2008. "An Exploration of Food Intolerance in the Primary Care Setting: The General Practitioner's Experience." *Social Science and Medicine* 67: 1038–1045.

Nhat Hanh, T. N., and L. Cheung. 2010. *Savor.* New York: HarperCollins.

Noble, E. P., R. E. Noble, T. Ritchie, K. Syndulko, M. C. Bohlman, L. A. Noble, Y. Zhang, R. S. Sparkes, and D. K. Grandy. 1994. "D2 Dopamine Receptor Gene and Obesity." *International Journal of Eating Disorders* 15: 205–217.

NPD Group. 2013. "Percentage of U.S. Adults Trying to Cut Down or Avoid Gluten in Their Diets Reaches New High in 2013, Reports NPD." http://www.npd.com/wps/portal/npd/us /news/press-releases/percentage-of-us-adults-trying-to-cut-down-or-avoid-gluten-in-their -diets-reaches-new-high-in-2013-reports-npd/. Accessed March 16, 2017.

Oliver, G., J. Wardle, E. L. Gibson. 2000. "Stress and Food Choice: A Laboratory Study." *Psychosomatic Medicine* 62: 853–865.

Ong, Z. Y., and B. S. Muhlhausler. 2011. "Maternal 'Junk Food' Feeding of rat Dams Alters Food Choices and Development of the Mesolimbic Pathway in Offspring." *FASEB Journal* 25: 2167–2179.

O'Reilly, G. A., L. Cook, D. Sprujit-Metz, and D. S. Black. 2014. Mindfulness-based interventions for obesity-related eating behaviours: A literature review. *Obesity Reviews* 15(6):453–61.

Parylak, S. L., G. F. Koob, and E. P. Zorrilla. 2011. "The Dark Side of Food Addiction." *Physiological Behavior* 104: 149–156.

Pelchat, M. L., A. Johnson, R. Chan, J. Valdez, and J. D. Ragland. 2004. "Images of Desire: Food Craving Activation During fMRI." *NeuroImage* 23: 1486–1493.

Perry, B. D. 2013. "Bonding and Attachment in Maltreated Children: Consequences of Emotional Neglect in Childhood." https://childtrauma.org/wp-content/uploads/2013/11/Bonding_13.pdf. Accessed March 16, 2017.

Pervanidou, P., and G. P. Chrousos. 2011. "Stress and Obesity/Metabolic Syndrome in Childhood and Adolescence." *International Journal of Pediatric Obesity* 6(Suppl 1): 21–28.

Philpott, W., and D. Kalita. 2000. *Brain Allergies: The Psychonutrient and Magnetic Connections.* Chicago: Keats Publishing.

Pinheiro, C. R., E. G. Moura, A. C. Manhaes, M. C. Fraga, S. Claudio-Neto, Y. Abreu-Villaça, E. Oliveira, and P. C. Lisboa. 2015. "Concurrent Maternal and Pup Postnatal Tobacco Smoke Exposure in Wistar Rats Changes Food Preferences and Dopaminergic Reward System Parameters in the Adult Male Offspring." *Neuroscience* 301: 178–192.

Pivarunas, B., and B. T. Conner. 2015. "Impulsivity and Emotion Dysregulation as Predictors of Food Addiction." *Eating Behaviors* 19: 9–14.

Puhl, R. M., C. A. Moss-Racusin, and B. Schwartz. 2007. "Internalization of Weight Bias: Implications for Binge Eating and Emotional Well-being." *Obesity (Silver Spring)* 15: 19–23.

Rodgers, R. F., S. J. Paxton, R. Massey, K. J. Campbell, E. H. Wertheim, H. Skouteris, and K. Gibbons. 2013. "Maternal Feeding Practices Predict Weight Gain and Obesogenic Eating Behaviors in Young Children: A Prospective Study." *International Journal of Behavioral Nutrition and Physical Activity* 10: 24.

Rolls, E. T., and C. McCabe. 2007. "Enhanced Affective Brain Representations of Chocolate in Cravers vs. Non-cravers." *European Journal of Neuroscience* 26: 1067–1076.

Rozenberg, S., J. J. Body, O. Bruyère, P. Bergmann, M. L. Brandi, C. Cooper, J. P. Devogelaer, E. Gielen, S. Goemaere, J. M. Kaufma, R. Rizzoli, and J. Y. Reginster. 2016. "Effects of

Dairy Products Consumption on Health: Benefits and Beliefs – A Commentary from the Belgian Bone Club and the European Society for Clinical and Economic Aspects of Osteoporosis, Osteoarthritis and Musculoskeletal Diseases." *Calcified Tissue International* 98: 1–17.

Rudd Center for Food Policy and Obesity. N.D. "Food Marketing." http://www.uconnrudd center.org/food-marketing. Accessed March 16, 2017.

Sapone, A., J. C. Bai, C. Ciacci, J. Dolinsek, P. H. Green, M. Hadjivassiliou, K. Kaukinen, K. Rostami, D. S. Sanders, M. Schumann, R. Ullrich, D. Villalta, U. Volta, C. Catassi, and A. Fasano. 2012. "Spectrum of Gluten-Related Disorders: Consensus on New Nomenclature and Classification." *BMC Medicine* 10: 13.

Segal, N. L., R. Feng, S. A. McGuire, D. B. Allison, and S. Miller. 2009. "Genetic and Environmental Contributions to Body Mass Index: Comparative Analysis of Monozygotic Twins, Dizygotic Twins and Same Age Unrelated Siblings." *International Journal of Obesity (London)* 33(1):37–41.

Shinohara, M., H. Mizushima, M. Hirano, K. Shioe, M. Nakazawa, Y. Hiejima, Y. Ono, and S. Kanba. 2004. "Eating Disorders with Binge Eating Behaviour Are Associated with the s Allele of the 3'-UTR VNTR Polymorphism of the Dopamine Transporter Gene." *Journal of Psychiatry and Neuroscience* 29: 134–137.

Siddiqui, S. V., U. Chatterjee, D. Kumar, A. Siddiqui, and N. Goyal. 2008. "Neuropsychology of Prefrontal Cortex." *Indian Journal of Psychiatry* 50: 202–208.

Simon, G. E., M. Von Korff, K. Saunders, D. L. Miglioretti, P. K. Crane, G. van Belle, and R. C. Kessler. 2006. "Association Between Obesity and Psychiatric Disorders in the US Adult Population." *Archives of General Psychiatry* 63: 824–830.

Sims, R., S. Gordon, W. Garcia, E. Clark, D. Monye, C. Callender, A. Campbell. 2008. "Perceived Stress and Eating Behaviors in a Community Sample of African Americans." *Eating Behaviors* 9: 137–142.

Sinha, R. 2008. "Chronic Stress, Drug Use, and Vulnerability to Addiction." *Annals of the New York Academy of Sciences* 1141: 105–130.

Sinha, R., H. C. Fox, K. A. Hong, K. Bergquist, Z. Bhagwagar, and K. M. Siedlarz. 2009. "Enhanced Negative Emotion and Alcohol Craving, and Altered Physiological Responses Following Stress and Cue Exposure in Alcohol Dependent Individuals." *Neuropsychopharmacology* 34: 1198–1208.

Small, D. M., M. Jones-Gotman, and A. Dagher. 2003. "Feeding-Induced Dopamine Release in Dorsal Striatum Correlates with Meal Pleasantness Ratings in Healthy Human Volunteers." *NeuroImage* 19: 1709–1715.

Soto, A. M., and C. Sonnenschein. 2010. "Environmental Causes of Cancer: Endocrine Disruptors as Carcinogens." *Nature Reviews Endocrinology* 6: 363–370.

Southwick, S., M. Vythilingam, and D. Charney. 2005. "The Psychobiology of Depression and Resilience to Stress: Implications for Prevention and Treatment." *Annual Review of Clinical Psychology* 1: 255–291.

Spring, B., K. Schneider, M. Smith, D. Kendzor, B. Appelhans, D. Hedeker, and S. Pagoto. 2008. "Abuse Potential of Carbohydrates for Overweight Carbohydrate Cravers." *Psychopharmacology (Berlin)* 197: 637–647.

Statista. 2016. "Statistics and Facts About Food Advertising." http://www.statista.com/topics /2223/food-advertising/. Accessed March 16, 2017.

Stice, E. 2002. "Risk and Maintenance Factors for Eating Pathology: A Meta-analytic Review." *Psychological Bulletin* 128: 825–848.

Stice, E., S. Spoor, C. Bohon, and D. M. Small. 2009a. "Relation Between Obesity and Blunted Striatal Response to Food Is Moderated by TaqlA A1 Allele." *Science* 322: 449–452.

Stice, E., S. Spoor, J. Ng, D. H. Zald. 2009b. "Relation of Obesity to Consummatory and Anticipatory Food Reward." *Physiology and Behavior* 97: 551–560.

Stice, E., S. Yokum, K. Blum, and C. Bohon. 2010. "Weight Gain Is Associated with Reduced Striatal Response to Palatable Food." *Journal of Neuroscience* 30: 13105–13109.

Stoeckel, L. E., R. E. Weller, E. W. Cook 3rd, D. B. Twieg, R. C. Knowlton, and J. E. Cox. 2008. "Widespread Reward-System Activation in Obese Women in Response to Pictures of High-Calorie Foods." *NeuroImage* 41: 636–647.

Su, X., H. Liang, W. Yuan, J. Olsen, S. Cnattingius, and J. Li. 2016. "Prenatal and Early Life Stress and Risk of Eating Disorders in Adolescent Girls and Young Women." *European Child and Adolescent Psychiatry* 25: 1245–1253.

Sun, J. 2010. "Vitamin D and Mucosal Immune Function." *Current Opinion in Gastroenterology* 26: 591–595.

Takser, L., D. Mergler, M. Baldwin, S. de Grosbois, A. Smargiassi, J. Lafond. 2005. "Thyroid Hormones in Pregnancy in Relation to Environmental Exposure to Organochlorine Compounds and Mercury." *Environmental Health Perspectives* 113: 1039–1045.

Talge, N. M., C. Neal, V. Glover, and Early Stress, Translational Research and Prevention Science Network. 2007. "Antenatal Maternal Stress and Long-Term Effects on Child Neurodevelopment: How and Why?" *Journal of Child Psychology and Psychiatry* 48: 245–261.

Teegarden, S. L., and T. L. Bale. 2007. "Decreases in Dietary Preference Produce Increased Emotionality and Risk for Dietary Relapse." *Biological Psychiatry* 61: 1021–1029.

Teicher, M. H. 2002. "Scars That Won't Heal: The Neurobiology of Child Abuse." *Scientific American* 296: 68–75.

Thomas, M. B., M. Hu, T. M. Lee, S. Bhatnagar, and J. B. Becker. 2009. "Sex-Specific Susceptibility to Cocaine in Rats with a History of Prenatal Stress." *Physiology and Behavior* 97: 270–277.

Torres, S. J., and C. A. Nowson. 2007. "Relationship Between Stress, Eating Behavior, and Obesity." *Nutrition* 23: 887–894.

Toschke, A. M., S. M. Montgomery, U. Pfeiffer, and R. von Kries. 2003. "Early Intrauterine Exposure to Tobacco-Inhaled Products and Obesity." *American Journal of Epidemiology* 158: 1068–1074.

Trasino, S. E., Y. D. Benoit, and L. J. Gudas. 2015. "Vitamin A Deficiency Causes Hyperglycemia and Loss of Pancreatic ß-Cell Mass." *The Journal of Biological Chemistry* 290: 1456–1473.

US Centers for Disease Control and Prevention. 2012. "Sexual Violence Facts at a Glance." http://www.cdc.gov/violenceprevention/pdf/sv-datasheet-a.pdf. Accessed March 16, 2017.

van der Kolk, B. A. 2005. "Developmental Trauma Disorder: Toward a Rational Diagnosis for Children with Complex Trauma Histories." *Psychiatric Annals* 35: 401–408.

Volkow, N. D., and C. P. O'Brien. 2007. "Issues for DSM-V: Should Obesity Be Included as a Brain Disorder?" *American Journal of Psychiatry* 164: 708–710.

Volkow, N. D., and R. A. Wise. 2005. "How Can Drug Addiction Help Us Understand Obesity?" *Nature Neuroscience* 8: 555–560.

Volkow, N. D., G.-J. Wang, J. S. Fowler, and F. Telang. 2008. "Overlapping Neuronal Circuits in Addiction and Obesity: Evidence of Systems Pathology." *Philosophical Transactions of the Royal Society of London. Series B, Biological Sciences* 363: 3191–3200.

Wade, T. D., and M. Tiggemann. 2013. "The Role of Perfectionism in Body Dissatisfaction." *Journal of Eating Disorders* 1: 2.

Wang, G.-J., A. Geliebter, N. D. Volkow , F. W. Telang, J. Logan, M. C. Jayne, K. Galanti, P. A. Selig, H. Han, W. Zhu, C. T. Wong, and J. S. Fowler. 2012. "Enhanced Striatal Dopamine Release During Food Stimulation in Binge Eating Disorder." *Obesity* 19: 1601–1608.

Wang, G.-J., N. D. Volkow, J. Logan, N. R. Pappas, C. T. Wong, W. Zhu, N. Netusil, and J. S. Fowler. 2001. "Brain Dopamine and Obesity." *Lancet* 357: 354–357.

Wang, G.-J., N. D. Volkow, F. W. Telang, M. C. Jayne, J. Ma, M. Rao, W. Zhu, C. T. Wong, N. R. Pappas, A. Geliebter, and J. S. Fowler. 2004. "Exposure to appetitive Food Stimuli Markedly Activates the Human Brain." *NeuroImage* 21: 1790–1797.

Warren, B. L., O. K. Sial, L. F. Alcantara, M. A. Greenwood, J. S. Brewer, J. P. Rozofsky, E. M. Parise, and C. A. Bolaños-Guzmán. 2014. "Altered Gene Expression and Spine Density in Nucleus Accumbens of Adolescent and Adult Male Mice Exposed to Emotional and Physical Stress." *Developmental Neuroscience* 36: 250–260.

Weaver, T. L., M. G. Griffin, and E. R. Mitchell. 2014. "Symptoms of Posttraumatic Stress, Depression and Body Image Distress in Female Victims of Physical and Sexual Assault: Exploring Integrated Responses." *Health Care for Women International* 35: 458–475.

Wilcox, C., and L. Brizendine. 2006. "For Women Only: Hormones May Prevent Addiction Relapse." *Current Psychiatry* 5: 40–52.

Williams, M., J. Teasdale, Z. Segal, and J. Kabat-Zinn. 2007. *The Mindful Way Through Depression.* New York: Guilford Press.

Wing, R. R., and S. Phelan. 2005. "Long-Term Weight Loss Maintenance." *American Journal of Clinical Nutrition* 82(1 Suppl): 222S–225S.

Witkiewitz, K., S. Bowen, H. Douglas, and S. H. Hsu. 2013. "Mindfulness-Based Relapse Prevention for Substance Craving." *Addictive Behaviors* 38: 1563–1571.

Wuttke, W., H. Jarry, and D. Seidlova-Wuttke. 2010. "Definition, Classification and Mechanism of Action of Endocrine Disrupting Chemicals." *Hormones (Athens)* 9: 9–15.

Yau, Y. H. C., and M. N. Potenza. 2013. "Stress and Eating Behaviors." *Minerva Endocrinologica* 38: 255–267.

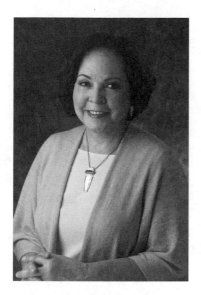

Carolyn Coker Ross, MD, MPH, is an internationally known author, speaker, expert, and pioneer in the use of integrative medicine for the treatment of eating disorders, obesity, and addictions. She is a graduate of Andrew Weil's Fellowship in Integrative Medicine program, and former head of the eating disorder program at internationally renowned Sierra Tucson. Ross is a consultant for treatment centers around the US, and author of three books, including *The Binge Eating and Compulsive Overeating Workbook* and her recent book, *The Emotional Eating Workbook*. Ross currently has a private practice in Denver, CO, and San Diego, CA, specializing in integrative medicine for treating eating disorders, addictions, mood and anxiety disorders, and obesity.

Ross is available for speaking engagements, and has spoken nationally and internationally on integrative medicine therapies for eating disorders and addictions. Her topics include integrative medicine for mental health issues, the treatment of food and body-image issues, and eating disorders and addictions. For more information, visit www.carolynrossmd.com/profes sional-services/speaking-engagements.

Ross also offers consulting services to help treatment centers build and incorporate eating disorder and addiction programs. For more information, visit www.carolynrossmd.com/profes sional-services/consultations.

The Anchor Program™

The Anchor Program™ is an international online coaching program for obesity, food addiction, and binge eating disorder that will help you take your recovery from food and eating addiction to the next level. You can work individually or in a group setting. For more information, visit www.findingyouranchor.com. I look forward to assisting you.

Reach Carolyn Ross by phone at 303-355-2445, or by e-mail at carolyn@carolynrossmd.com.

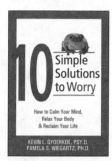
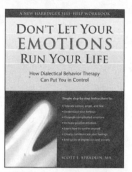
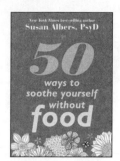
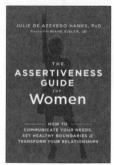
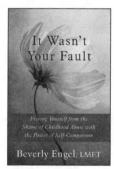
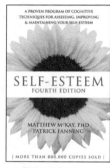 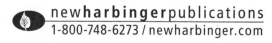

Register your **new harbinger** titles for additional benefits!

When you register your **new harbinger** title—purchased in any format, from any source—you get access to benefits like the following:

- Downloadable accessories like printable worksheets and extra content

- Instructional videos and audio files

- Information about updates, corrections, and new editions

Not every title has accessories, but we're adding new material all the time.

Access free accessories in 3 easy steps:

1. Sign in at NewHarbinger.com (or **register** to create an account).

2. Click on **register a book**. Search for your title and click the **register** button when it appears.

3. Click on the **book cover or title** to go to its details page. Click on **accessories** to view and access files.

That's all there is to it!

If you need help, visit:

NewHarbinger.com/accessories

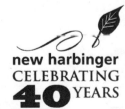

new harbinger
CELEBRATING
40 YEARS